THE TIRED CHILD

How Sleep and Sleep Breathing
Can Change Your Child's Life

THE TIRED CHILD

Dr. Meghna Dassani

Copyright © 2023 by Dr. Meghna Dassani

All rights reserved. No part of this book may be used or reproduced in any manner whatsoever without prior written consent of the author, except as provided by the United States of America copyright law.

Published by Best Seller Publishing®, St. Augustine, FL
Best Seller Publishing® is a registered trademark.
Printed in the United States of America.
ISBN: 978-1-959840-47-3

This publication is designed to provide accurate and authoritative information with regard to the subject matter covered. It is sold with the understanding that the publisher is not engaged in rendering legal, accounting, or other professional advice. If legal advice or other expert assistance is required, the services of a competent professional should be sought. The opinions expressed by the author in this book are not endorsed by Best Seller Publishing® and are the sole responsibility of the author rendering the opinion.

For more information, please write:
Best Seller Publishing®
53 Marine Street
St. Augustine, FL 32084
or call 1 (626) 765-9750
Visit us online at: www.BestSellerPublishing.org

BOOK REVIEWS

"In *The Tired Child*, Dr. Meghna Dassani does an incredible job depicting how poor sleep is the culprit, negatively impacting our children in a multitude of ways. She has a unique way of connecting with readers and explaining the science of sleep in a digestible manner.

Dr. Dassani makes it very clear that we MUST be our children's advocates, getting to root causes instead of treating symptoms with bandaids that are bound to fail. By doing so, we are giving our children the ability to unlock their fullest potential, thrive, and grow into the very best versions of themselves."

- Brittny Sciarra-Murphy, RDH, BS, MAS™, QOM®, COM®

"Dr. Dassani's new book offers a great insight into why a child may be struggling with normal activities, even after having multiple specialists evaluate the child unable to determine an exact cause for the symptoms. Dr. Dassani makes it easy to understand and follow along to gain basic knowledge of the importance of sleep, breathing, and airway. For parents struggling to find the "why" to the symptoms, this book will show how important quality sleep and breathing is for each child."

- Amanda Sharp DDS

"Dr. Dassani does it again! What a fabulous book. As a dentist and mom of children with sleep disordered breathing, I can not only empathize with the histories of this book but understand what is going on. Dr. Dassani explains the signs and symptoms of Sleep disordered breathing (SDB) in a simple yet powerful way. SDB is becoming a pandemic. A lot of signs and symptoms are being mis-diagnosed or not given the importance they deserve. If you, mama, feel that the diagnosis and/or treatment given by your health care provider is not correct or they are missing something, follow your gut and seek a second opinion. As a mom, I encourage this to my patients. Don't let anyone brush away your concerns. You, your children and your family deserve it. Problems with sleep breathing affect the whole family. Someone needs to be that advocate. After reading this book: "You will be that advocate!"

- Norma Cortez, DDS

"Dr. Dassani's book is prioritizing the message of healthy sleep in our children. This is something not talked about enough and has deleterious effects. This is a wonderful eye-opening resource that takes relatable scenarios to clinically frame the issues."

- Autumn R. Henning, MS, CCC-SLP, COM, IBCLC

"Every parent and practitioner needs to read this book! Dr. Dassani clearly explains the literal life changing impact adequate sleep can have on a child and their growth and development. With research to back her findings, stories that every struggling parent can relate to, and answers that could take you years to find on your own, this is a road map for healthy kids and parents to follow. Start HERE!"

- Michelle Jorgensen DDS

"Dr. Dassani has a unique way of taking a complex subject like sleep, and presenting it in a simple manner that is easy for both professionals and patients to understand. Her use of real life stories helps the reader identify and relate to symptoms their child or patient may be experiencing. This book draws attention to the symptoms a lot of children are experiencing today, and how a lack of understanding about pediatric sleep apnea is resulting in our children being either misdiagnosed with ADHD or being labeled as difficult. It also makes us aware of the long term effects of untreated sleep apnea in children. If we want a healthy society long term, we need to address and treat sleep issues in our kids. I highly recommend this book not only to dentists and parents, but also to all healthcare professionals who treat children in their practice."

- Nimisha Somaiya DDS

"Dr. Meghna Dassani is, simply put, an amazing teacher. Reading her books on Sleep Disordered Breathing (SDB) has opened my eyes to the many possibilities out there for a more nuanced planning of patient treatment. Specifically with children, dentists are at the forefront of treating them at an age where different techniques can be implemented with profound life-lasting results. Dr. Dassani's careful weaving of the issues we face alongside our pediatric patients makes this book an absolute treasure. It can be used as a Guide for not only dentists, but for parents, teachers, families, and other healthcare professionals. As a relative "newbie" to the world of Sleep Disordered Breathing, I have found Dr. Dassani's words to be very precise, understandable, but even more importantly, relatable. She humanizes what our patients are going through, thereby creating a sense of urgency that allows one to easily take the lessons learned in each chapter and apply them the following day. And once SDB issues are noticed, it's hard to unsee them, especially in our youngest patients. Once we understand the issues our patients are facing, we become better equipped to guide our patients to a better, healthier future. I highly recommend this book for anyone who is looking for a better understanding of SDB as it pertains to pediatrics. I know that I will be using it for many years to come to help navigate the world of Pediatric Sleep Disordered Breathing."

- Shailee S. Patel, DDS

"Dr. Meghna Dassani has made it easy for parents to truly understand why sleep is so important and how poor sleep may be impacting their children in major ways. Sometimes it feels like the world has gone crazy with the focus on treating symptoms with bandaids. If your children are struggling but no one has taken the time to thoroughly assess them for the first foundations of health, breathing and sleep, this book will empower you to find the help they need!"

- Tara Erson, DMD, IBCLC, D. ABDSM

"Dr. Dassani does it again! *The Tired Child* goes searching for mother's hearts that are broken for their kids. It's for those strong mothers who have been tirelessly looking for answers without a clear understanding of their child's symptoms.

As a professional in this field, we know that children will react and adapt differently to their disordered breathing during the day and at night. This book connects caregivers to the answers they were looking for, all in an easily digestible format. Thank you for taking the time to write this book Dr. Dassani! Our lost sleepless children are waiting to be found."

- Renata Nehme, RDH, BSDH, COM®

"I'm a mom of 2 and a Board Certified Pediatric Dentist. For 3 years, I watched my own son struggle due to what I perceived as a sleep disorder. His 'issues' were brushed off as he wasn't demonstrating extreme behaviors but he chronically had a cold, was at a low weight percentile category, and his sleep was extremely restless. My parent intuition told me something was wrong. It wasn't until I took Dr. Dassani's Course that I learned, my assumptions were exactly correct. Thanks to her guidance, my son is a different, healthy, happy, well rested child and I am a different provider for my patients. Sleep matters. *The Tired Child* should be on every parent's (and provider's) bookshelf."

- Dr. Jonelle Anamelechi

"So many children are failed by the lack of knowledge in Sleep Disordered Breathing and the effects on their development. Unfortunately, most physicians are ill prepared to diagnose the underlying cause of a child's symptoms and therefore treat the symptoms while the child continues to suffer and the parents feel helpless. Dr Meghna Dassani has made it her life's mission to bring awareness of sleep breathing and sleep loss to the medical community and to parents looking for answers. This book will give you, the parent, the answers to identify the cause of your child's symptoms and how to get the help your child needs. You will finally be able to help your child sleep soundly and truly become the best version of themselves. This is a book that you will reference often and will help you be able to seek out the medical professionals that have the experience to recognize the issues at hand and help your child get on the right path to health. This book will also raise awareness among the medical and dental professionals so that they can recognize sleep loss in a child and either treat the cause or be able to refer the child to the correct professionals."

- Anna Pollatos DDS

"As a dental professional who treats all ages in my practice, this book by Dr. Dassani provides parents/caretakers the most clear and comprehensive correlations in early sleep screening and intervention. I can not wait to share this with my patients so they can continue to find solutions to their children's sleep and behavior problems!"

- Sapna Amin-Makan DDS

"A revelation for desperate parents who know there is something wrong with their child but no one seems to give them answers. Dr. Dassani lays it all out for us clinicians and parents connecting the dots to the silent epidemic of sleep disorder breathing."

- Marisabel Olivera, DMD (Pediatric Dentist)

"As parents, we can tell when something isn't right with our child, and we will exhaust all avenues trying to figure out how to correct it. Unfortunately, there are few options available to treat children who present with ADHD, colic, fussy eating, bed wetting; kids who fight sleep, snore, or struggle with nightmares. We are told they'll grow out of the problem; it's normal. Our children are given labels – ADHD, dyslexic, ASD, or just… difficult; challenging. Dr. Dassani educates parents on the reasons underlying sleep, what constitutes normal sleep cycles, and what happens when those cycles are broken. She makes it easy to understand why our sleep deprived children struggle. Dr. Dassani provides us with insights and hope for why and how our tired children can get the rest they need to thrive and grow to become their best selves. She does so gently and without blame, empowering parents to seek the help they need."

- Dr. Preeya Genz

For Sweta. My sister. My ride or die.
The best friend a girl can ask for.

CONTENTS

Book Reviews v
Acknowledgements xvii
Introduction: What is Wrong with My Child?. xix

CHAPTER 1: The Sleep-Deprived Child. 1
    Ryan's Story. 1
    Cleo's Story 1
    Willow's Story 2
    A 'Cure' that Doesn't Address Sleep
        Breathing is No Cure at All. 3
    Why Are Pediatric Sleep Issues Suddenly
        Such a Big Thing?. 5
    If My Child is Sleep-Deprived, Why Isn't She Tired? 7
    The Short-term Effects of Sleep Loss on Children. 8
    The Long-term Effects of Sleep Loss on Children 9

CHAPTER 2: Why Kids Need Sleep 11
    The Biology of Sleep in Children 11
    The Structure of Sleep 12
    The Five Sleep Stages and What They Do for Children. . 13
    The 5 Stages Combined Make One Sleep Cycle 15

    Circadian Rhythms 16
    Sleep Changes As People Grow. 17
    What Do All These Patterns Do For My Child? 18
    Meet Jackson, The Child Who Gets Enough Sleep 20
    Change the Sleep, Change the Child's Life. 21

CHAPTER 3: Sleep Thieves. 23
    Modern Living is Anti-Sleep 23
    Some Kids Are Born Bad Sleepers 27
    What Your Kid Eats Can Change How They Sleep. 31
    Sometimes, the Inability to Sleep is All in Their Mind. . .34
    Illnesses, Allergies, and Asthma 35
    When The Airway is Blocked .36

CHAPTER 4: Airway Up Close 41
    The Upper Airway and Its Role During Sleep 41
    What Good Are Noses and Sinuses? 42
    How Do Kids Get UARS or OSA?. 45
    How Tongue Tie Impacts the Development
        of the Airways, and Other Parts of Life Too!. 47
    How Does Tongue Tie Affect Growth and
        Development? 48
    Why Tongue Ties Don't Get Treated in Infancy. 51

CHAPTER 5: Restore Sleep, Save the Child 53
    I'm Worried About My Kid. Who Can I Talk To? 53
    What Will My Child's Diagnostic Process for
        OSA Look Like? 56
    What are the Most Common Treatments if My Child is
        Diagnosed with OSA?. 59

CHAPTER 6: Palates, Tongues, and Tonsils. 63

    What Are Tonsils and Adenoids Anyway?. 63
    What is T&A surgery?. 64
    What Happens When A Child Gets T&A Surgery?. 65
    Are There Any Long-Term Effects of T&A surgery?. . . .65
    Why Do Tonsils and Adenoids Swell?. 66
    How Does Mouth Breathing Contribute to Swelling? . . .67
    Why is My Child a Mouth-Breather Anyway? 68
    An Ounce of Prevention. 70
    Evaluate and Treat Tongue-Ties First! 71
    Why Can Fixing Tongue-Tie Fix OSA? 74
    What Comes Next After a Tongue-Tie is Released?. 75
    What if We Try All of These Things, and the Tonsils and
        Adenoids Are Still A Problem?. 79

CHAPTER 7: Supporting Healthy Sleep at Home. 81

    Screen Time, and How to Limit It 81
    What to Do About All the CFL and LED Lights 83
    Steps to Creating Allergy-Friendly Sleeping Areas 84
    Foods and Supplements that Support Healthy Sleep 86
    Reset Your Kid's Circadian Rhythm. 89
    The Best Exercises for Sleep 89
    Destress Before Bedtime 90
    What About Bedwetting?. 91
    We Were Doing Great—Until We Hit the Teens!. 92
    You're Well On Your Way to Great Sleep for Your Kids .94

CHAPTER 8: Congratulations! You're a Kids' Sleep Expert. . .95

APPENDIX 1: Resources for Finding Help for Your Child. . .97

APPENDIX 2: Book Club Discussion Guide 99

    Introduction and Chapter 1. 99
    Chapter 2. 100
    Chapter 3. 100
    Chapter 4. 101
    Chapter 5. 101
    Chapter 6. 102
    Chapter 7. 102
    Chapter 8. 103

APPENDIX 3: Sources and Further Reading. 105

    Articles. 105
    Other Reading. 107

APPENDIX 4: Worksheets 109

    My Healthy Sleep Plan 109
    My Sleep Team 110

ACKNOWLEDGEMENTS

After *Airway Is Life*, I promised myself I was done. I was convinced I had shared all I could with those seeking answers to their family's sleep issues. But a little voice in the back of my head kept asking, "What about the kids? Who is going to be their voice?"

Add to it all the children and their parents who trust me with their sleep and health every single day. All the stories. All the worry that parents bring me everyday.

At some point, my girls have been those kids. Sleep deprived, tired, exhausted.

And the kids I get to claim as my own...those of my team members and friends and everyone else in my life.

That is how *The Tired Child* was born. I hope it gives some answers to those seeking them as I was when I was a new mom.

No endeavor is complete without thanking the amazing humans in my life.

My girls, Nandini and Maadhvi...you are my reason for everything I do. My world is bright because of you in it.

My sister and parents... you constantly encourage me to aim high and admonish me when I sell myself short or allow the doubts to seep in .

Christina...for making my dreams yours and putting up with my madness. Words aren't enough....

Vanna… you define sunshine. Thank you for sharing your light.
My patients and their parents who trust me with their health. Thank you for allowing me to love your families like my own. This book is yours. For you.

Eternally grateful.

INTRODUCTION
WHAT IS WRONG WITH MY CHILD?

You're at the playground, and you can feel the stress building. While other kids play nicely, your child has no resilience. Every bumped elbow is a major meltdown. When she was younger, she was the biter. Everyone tells you it's just a discipline problem, but no one else is working this hard to keep their child happy at the playground.

You're at work and the phone rings. You check the caller ID and sigh. It's the school. You're going to have to take this one. Your son hasn't turned in any work all year and keeps distracting the other kids. You've already taken him for an evaluation, it's not ADHD. You just don't know how to reach him or motivate him. He's such a smart kid, but he's failing.

Your kid loves soccer. She practices at home all the time. She's not bad at it either, but put her in a game and it's like her brain is broken. She's the team space cadet. She never notices where the ball is, no matter how much everyone screams. It's like she's in her own world, so she spends a lot of time on the bench. She's starting to lose her love for the game because she's just 'no good at it.'

It's bedtime, and you go through the routine and get everyone to sleep by nine. It never makes a difference. Mornings are terrible because your children just can't seem to wake up and get moving. Every day there are tears, complaints about headaches, and dawdling. They're getting as much sleep as the pediatrician recommended, so why are they always so tired?

You're the parent. You know your child better than anyone else. And you know that there's something wrong with them, despite teachers and doctors suggesting that it's just a problem with scheduling and discipline. It can't be normal for a child to live this way!

You're right. It's not normal. There's something wrong with your child. They're not a bad kid. They want to socialize, succeed at school, and get up in the morning. No one likes getting in trouble all the time or seeing a C on a test. Your child isn't failing at things because they want to, or because they are stubborn. They are failing because something in their body or brain is keeping them from succeeding. It's time to find the underlying cause of their problems and treat it.

For many American children, that problem is sleep.

Our nation is facing an epidemic of disturbed sleep. It's not just overweight, middle-aged adults. Sleep issues run through our society. Many physicians aren't trained to recognize them or to detect the physical issues contributing to poor sleep. Right now, problems with sleep are disrupting your children's lives and threatening their futures.

By learning about sleep in children and taking steps to correct your family's sleep, you can change their lives.

In this book, you'll learn how to spot the symptoms of sleep disorders in children and how those disorders lead to changes in behavior, physical and mental health, and learning capabilities. You'll learn how sleep is supposed to work, and how healthy sleep supports your child's physical, intellectual, social, and emotional growth. Then, we'll do a deep dive into the various causes of sleep deprivation in kids, and ways to treat them so that you can give your child a good night's sleep. Finally, you'll learn how to support healthy sleep at home. This book works both as something you read straight through and as a reference guide as you try to improve your family's health. How you use it will depend on your needs.

Together, we can change your children's sleep and change their lives.

CHAPTER 1
THE SLEEP-DEPRIVED CHILD

Ryan's Story

Ryan was a genuinely difficult kid. By the time he was two, he had cut out all naps and didn't sleep more than four hours a night. His parents and other caregivers found him exhausting. The child was driven by a motor and tore up everything around him.

Discipline never worked. Sleep routines didn't work. By first grade, he had an ADHD diagnosis. His parents agreed to try stimulants. They made him worse. Now he had anxiety on top of his ADHD, and he was aggressive. They tried one medicine after another, but nothing treated his ADHD.

Ryan's mother began to wonder if maybe the ADHD was a symptom, not the cause, of all of her son's behavioral issues.

Cleo's Story

Cleo had been a cranky, colicky infant. She nursed constantly, until her mother's nipples were cracked and broken, but never seemed to get enough food. Weaning her onto a bottle seemed to help a bit, but she was still slow to grow, gassy, and prone to vomit.

As she got older, the stomach issues seemed to improve, but she had a noticeable speech impediment. At school, she was pegged as a space cadet. She was a conscientious kid but was still wetting the bed in Kindergarten. Her speech, bladder, and attention issues were starting to affect her self-esteem. Her parents and teachers were at a loss. Cleo was a sweet kid, but she struggled so much. What could anyone do for her?

WILLOW'S STORY

Willow had always been prone to allergies, sinus infections, and earaches. She was on a ton of allergy medicines, but it seemed like nothing could keep her nose clear. Over time, she'd fallen into the habit of mouth-breathing.

She was also an incredibly finicky eater, and everyone remembered her as a 'chokey kid.' If a food's texture wasn't exactly right, she had trouble chewing and swallowing. So many meals ended in gagging that her parents had gotten into the habit of putting the trash can next to her chair so she'd have somewhere to spit out those big lumps of food.

No one had ever made the connection between her sinus issues and her eating issues, so her parents just gave her vitamin supplements and hoped she'd eventually grow out of her problems.

These three children are very different, they are three faces of the same underlying problem. Their parents can tell something is wrong with their children, but they're unsure what to do about it. None of the normal solutions seem to help. Do their children simply have to struggle forever? Why can't they find a cure?

There is a cure available for children like Ryan, Cleo, and Willow. Each of these children is experiencing a disruption of a biological process that is essential for human functioning and flourishing. Each of these children has been seen by multiple specialists. They've been poked, prodded, and medicated. But until that underlying issue is identified and treated, they will continue to suffer.

What one issue links all three of these children?
Sleep breathing.

A 'Cure' that Doesn't Address Sleep Breathing is No Cure at All

Why haven't the specialists been able to cure Ryan, Cleo, and Willow? Because their treatments focus on the strange and disruptive symptoms the children are presenting, but not on the underlying cause that unites those symptoms.

When a child's sleep breathing is disrupted, their sleep is disrupted. When a child's sleep is disrupted, their life falls to pieces. Good sleep is necessary to:

- Regulate the parts of the brain that handle self-control, mood, and social skills
- Consolidate memories and learning
- Release the hormones necessary for healthy growth
- Support the immune system
- Fight inflammation
- Ensure a happy, healthy child

The underlying conditions that most commonly affect sleep breathing in children also affect:

- Sinus function
- Chewing and swallowing
- Speech
- Posture

- Daytime breathing
- Lung function
- Digestion

To cure the child, you must fix the sleep breathing and the underlying issues that caused the breathing problems in the first place.

For children like Ryan, Cleo, and Willow, their first weeks of real, restful, healthy sleep are life-changing. Parents report that the rest of the world can finally see the good things about their children. Kids make huge leaps in learning, energy levels, and social skills.

Since 2012, the American Academy of Pediatrics has recommended that any child who shows signs of sleep disturbances or behavior problems should be referred for sleep testing. However, very few practices actually follow these recommendations. Why?

Because parents aren't willing to hear the news about sleep and children, pediatric sleep labs are rare and often overbooked, and the most common treatments for pediatric sleep apnea are expensive and difficult. For many practitioners and parents, waiting to see if the child outgrows the problem seems like the safest step. Unfortunately, waiting for sleep issues to resolve on their own can result in permanent damage to the child.

Every year that sleep breathing issues continue can result in lasting harm to a child's learning, self-esteem, and physical health.

If you want to save the child, you have to save their sleep first. There are practitioners out there who will address child sleep issues and help your child. To find them, you have to educate yourself and be ready to advocate for your child. You can become an expert, and get your child the help they need.

Why Are Pediatric Sleep Issues Suddenly Such a Big Thing?

There are a few reasons that sleep issues seem to be impacting children today more than they impacted children in the past.

The Twenty-first Century Lifestyle

One reason children struggle with healthy sleep is our lifestyle. Today, children get less time outside during the sunny parts of the day, spend more time on screens, and have less time to unwind before bed. All of these changes affect the brain's ability to settle down for healthy, healing sleep.

While some kids can adjust and still fall asleep easily, more sensitive kids are unable to settle into sleep quickly. Their brain patterns are affected and their sleep is just not as healthy or restful.

Increased Awareness

One reason parents are hearing more about childhood sleep issues now is that we have a greater understanding of pediatric sleep and brain development. In the past, a child with sleep issues may have been labeled "just a bad kid." But now we understand that most young children *want* to behave well, some just *can't*.

We also realize that conditions like sleep apnea present differently in children and that sleep apnea isn't limited to children who struggle with obesity. *Thin, active kids can also have major problems with their sleep.*

Finally, there is now an established standard of care for children with sleep problems. In the past, it wasn't diagnosed as much because all physicians could do was wait for the child to grow out of the problem. Today, we understand brain chemistry, oral-facial development, and breathing much better, so we can treat children who were previously untreatable.

A Change in the Standard of Care

Finally, a major change in the standard of care for infants has increased sleep breathing problems, and other issues, in older children.

For much of human history, the standard of care was to "clip" tongue and lip ties at birth. These pieces of tissue can keep the tongue, lips, and cheeks from working efficiently to nurse, speak, eat and breathe.

When bottle feeding became more prevalent, the clipping stopped, because the most obvious and immediate problems were limited to breastfeeding. Now, if an infant struggles with a tongue or lip-tie, it can be difficult for a parent to get help unless the child is failing to thrive.

However, tongue ties cause big problems in older children too. During sleep, the tongue must rest on the palate to keep the airway open. When a child has an unrevised tongue tie, the tongue can fall back into their throat and restrict air supply.

In addition, during infancy and childhood, the tongue normally acts as a natural palate expander. The palate is not just the roof of the mouth, it's also the floor of the nasal cavity. When the tongue pushes against the palate during sleep, it widens it, so that the nasal cavity becomes larger and less prone to blockage.

When a child has a high narrow palate resulting from a life-long tongue tie or due to a developmental condition, the nose becomes easily blocked. The child breathes through his mouth and inflames his throat, tonsils, and adenoids. They swell and narrow the airway. Then the tongue blocks it a little more, and Boom! The child cannot get enough air to sleep well.

In the pediatric sleep world, the change in tongue tie standards has resulted in an epidemic of older kids who can't breathe at night.

If My Child is Sleep-Deprived, Why Isn't She Tired?

One reason parents, teachers, and physicians often miss the symptoms of a sleepless child is that children react to sleep issues in unique ways.

Adults with sleep breathing problems appear tired, depressed, achy, and forgetful. They act the way that other adults expect an exhausted person to act. Children *can* display these symptoms, but they can also:

- Wet the bed because, without healthy sleep, the body doesn't concentrate urine at night

- Thrash around in sleep, changing position and tangling up the sheets and blankets

- Snore, gasp, cough, or choke in the night

- Display an open-mouthed posture during the day

- Become hyperactive to help themselves stay awake and alert

- Lose emotional control so that they throw tantrums, act aggressive, or melt-down

- Have night terrors and never grow out of them

- Have trouble focusing that translates to trouble with school and time management

- Develop anxiety because a sleepless brain can't meet the demands of their lives

- Have trouble learning and retaining new information

- Have frequent upper respiratory infections and seem to always be sick

- Struggle at sports and have trouble learning new physical skills
- Forget where they are in a task and constantly wander off task

These symptoms cluster differently in each child, but if you notice that several of them fit your child, it's time to take a close look at sleep.

Remember, these kids are not bad kids. They are kids that are not getting enough of something ***essential to human life and flourishing.***

Children are not small adults.

Remember, one reason that this list of symptoms is so different from the symptoms of adults with similar issues is that children are in a period of rapid growth and development.

Much of that development is happening in their brain, and when they don't sleep well, they lose out on development.

When you see an adult who slowly developed obstructive sleep apnea as they aged, they have the benefits of years of normal sleep, growth, and learning.

For kids, sleep issues are literally stunting their mental growth. You cannot expect them to react to sleep loss as an adult would.

THE SHORT-TERM EFFECTS OF SLEEP LOSS ON CHILDREN

In the short term, the effects of sleep loss can be reversible. Children who are not getting a full night's sleep may have stunted growth or, alternatively, struggle with obesity. That's because one role of sleep is controlling the hormones that the child needs to grow and heal.

They may wet the bed because their brain isn't deeply asleep and so the body doesn't concentrate urine.

They may have trouble learning new skills, both academic ones like reading and math, and physical ones like dribbling, swimming, or driving.

They may be more emotional and have a harder time getting along with family and friends. They may be more impulsive and disobedient.

They might have frequent headaches, have eating issues, and be generally 'off' a lot of the time.

The good news is that with proper identification and treatment, we can get these kids back on their developmental path, and they can catch up. They can grow normally, learn normally, and socialize normally. They can start living a healthier, happier life, If only they get treatment.

When these kids fly under the radar for years, things get more serious.

The Long-term Effects of Sleep Loss on Children

When a child goes without sleep long-term, the situation becomes worse.

A lifetime of respiratory illness takes a toll on the body, and they're at increased risk for asthma.

Chronic exposure to stress hormones from a brain that isn't getting enough sleep leads to obesity, type II diabetes, high blood pressure, cardiac issues, chronic pain, and autoimmune problems.

They've fallen years behind in school, they can't focus, and they can't catch up or reach their potential.

Their habitual open-mouthed posture has affected their facial development and their dental health, leading to life-long pain and other problems.

They're sleepy drivers, and that makes them accident-prone drivers. These kids are totaling cars, getting tickets, and sometimes getting severely injured in auto accidents.

After years of being labeled a "bad kid" or a "dumb kid" by peers and adults, their self-esteem is in terrible shape. Eventually, depression and anxiety set in and these kids just stop trying. Why bother? They can't learn anyway and they always mess up every social situation. Some of these kids will try to self-medicate with drugs or alcohol, and we'll lose them to addiction. Others will become self-harming. The years of problems at home and school, combined with the years of lost brain development, take a toll.

All of these outcomes are preventable. We need to get these kids diagnosed and treated so that they can live their best lives. What your child needs is an educated advocate, someone who understands the role of sleep, what can go wrong, and how to find treatment.

By the time you finish this book, **You Will Be That Advocate.**

CHAPTER 2
WHY KIDS NEED SLEEP

To understand what's going on with your child, you need to first understand what healthy sleep for children looks like.

Sleep is essential for our bodies. It's how we heal, grow, learn and learn. Sleep regulates our systems, gives us time to work out the puzzles in our lives, and relieves stress. We all need uninterrupted, healthy sleep. And kids need a lot more of that healthy sleep than adults do.

This chapter is a basic science lesson on what sleep does. It's focused on pediatric sleep science, but much of what we'll discuss applies to adults too. Sleep science is new, fascinating, and exciting. It's the key to living longer, healthier, and more fulfilling lives. Once you understand how many good things sleep does for your child, you'll become passionate about ensuring that they get good sleep.

THE BIOLOGY OF SLEEP IN CHILDREN

Have you ever watched a baby or toddler sleep? At first, their eyes open at every sound, they move and react, and it's possible to wake them up if you have to. Then, they go totally limp, like a ragdoll. You can't wake them up, even if you move them from car to crib or bustle around the room.

If you watch them long enough, you may notice a change in breathing and movement that tells you that they're dreaming. Maybe you'll even see them smile or laugh in their sleep. Eventually, as their time for sleeping ends, you can see them grow responsive again. They're waking up, and if you want them to sleep long you'll have to be quiet and keep others from disturbing them.

You've just observed your child going through multiple stages of sleep. Each of these stages has a different job and provides different benefits. All healthy humans go through these same stages, but we spend different times in each stage at different ages.

THE STRUCTURE OF SLEEP

Healthy human sleep follows patterns. As we sleep, we move through 5 stages of sleep. When a person moves through a group of stages, that's one sleep cycle. We need multiple completed sleep cycles every night.

Our cycles look different at the beginning of the night than at the end. This is why cutting your sleep short on either end, or sleeping at a different time of day than your usual time, can make your sleep less restful and healthy.

Everyone has their own pattern of when they feel wide awake and when they feel sleepy. This is their circadian rhythm. Circadian rhythms are one reason that some kids are clearly early birds, and others are night owls. You can bump the circadian rhythm a little bit earlier or later, but big changes just result in disrupted, unhealthy sleep.

The Five Sleep Stages and What They Do for Children

Adults and children have the same stages of sleep, but these cycles have different jobs at different points in our lives. This is one reason why a sleep-deprived kid and a sleep-deprived adult may look like they have two totally different conditions.

Scientists learn about sleep stages and what they do for the body by studying sleeping children in labs. They measure their brainwaves and take blood and urine samples to see what the body is doing and how their hormones are changing.

They also study children with poor sleep. They can use brainwaves to see which stages of sleep are disrupted for the child. Then they can see which life functions are disrupted in children with certain sleep problems.

Sleep science is still a young science. New discoveries are coming out every day! What follows is the current state of the science in Summer 2022. Wait a year or so, and we may learn even more things that healthy sleep does for your child's brain and body!

Stage 0: Being Awake

Why do we count wakefulness as one of the sleep stages? First of all, every sleeper was first awake. Second of all, after a sleep cycle ends, people often wake up briefly. If your child can resettle quickly, you might not notice these periods of wakefulness. However, if your child wakes up and is thirsty, scared, lonely, or chatty, you're well aware that "sleeping through the night" is a misnomer.

For infants, this periodic waking can literally be a lifesaver. It ensures that nursing infants get enough nutrition, and it even helps prevent Sudden Infant Death Syndrome. (SIDS). Some older children may wake up, get a drink, read for a bit, and go back to sleep halfway through the night. As long as waking is only happening after a completed cycle and the child can resettle to complete their full night of sleep, it's a normal part of being human.

Stage 1: Nodding off

As the brain drifts off to sleep, a child's breathing and heart rate slow down. Their body temperature gets lower. Their brain waves start to slow down and become less reactive. Their thoughts get confused and they may suddenly startle and jerk back awake.

You can watch a child literally "Nod off" in their car seat, in front of the TV, or even at the dinner table. Once the brain is sure that they are in a safe place for sleeping, they'll slip into the next stage of sleep.

Stage 2: Light Sleep

Stage 2 sleep is also called NREM sleep, meaning Non-Dreaming sleep. This light NREM sleep is the kind that children and adults experience during short naps, and it's the gateway to other sleep stages. In Stage two sleep, brain activity slows except for occasional bursts of energy called sleep spindles.

Scientists aren't completely sure what these sleep spindles do, but they appear to have a role in enhancing memory, sorting and consolidating new information, and insulating the sleeping brain from the sounds, smells, and feelings in the environment.

Stages 3 and 4: Deep Sleep

Sleep Scientists argue about whether deep sleep is better described as two stages or one, and about where the division between stages 3 and 4 falls.

What they do know is that when deep sleep is healthy sleep, the body goes limp. Breathing is totally regular and rhythmic. The brain waves organize into what scientists call Delta Waves or slow wave sleep. During deep sleep, the body grows and heals itself. The brain rewires itself. This is why kids seem to sleep so much more when they're having a growth spurt or about to hit a new developmental milestone.

When a child is failing to grow, missing milestones, and having trouble bouncing back from illness and accidents, they may not be getting the full benefit of deep sleep.

Stage 5: REM Sleep

After a period of deep sleep, the brain moves back to light sleep. But then, instead of going back to deep sleep, it often enters a period of REM sleep, or rapid eye movement sleep. This is when people dream. These dreams can help them cope with social and emotional problems, navigate the world, and solve problems creatively.

THE 5 STAGES COMBINED MAKE ONE SLEEP CYCLE

A sleep cycle is a period of time where someone goes through all the stages of sleep. People have multiple sleep cycles every night. Children have more than adults because their sleep cycles are shorter and they spend more time asleep.

As the night progresses, your child's sleep cycles change. At first, they have longer periods of deep sleep and only very short periods of REM sleep. In the early part of the night, your child is healing and growing.

As morning approaches, these cycles change. The periods of deep sleep get shorter as the periods of REM sleep get longer.

When a child goes to bed late, they may miss out on some of their deep sleep, but get sufficient REM sleep. If the child is woken up too early, they may get most of their deep sleep, but miss most of their REM sleep.

People need both deep sleep and REM sleep to thrive so, for healthy sleep, it's important to get kids to bed on time and let them sleep as long as they need to in the morning.

Circadian Rhythms

Circadian rhythms are the pattern your brain and body follow during the day. Your temperature, wakefulness level, and hunger levels all rise and fall every day. Your Circadian rhythm determines when the body releases hormones so that you get ready for bed.

Sunlight has a big factor on Circadian rhythm. Absorbing the rays of the sun through the eyes sends signals to your brain about what time of day it is. In the evening, the red light of dusk and sunset triggers a chemical release that tells your body it's time for bed.

Without these cues from the sun, the brain and body get confused. People who suffer from blindness and people who have stayed underground in darkness for long periods of time find that their circadian rhythms often get 'off' and no longer follow a standard day.

Too much artificial light, especially the blue light from certain lightbulbs and the screens on electronic devices, can also interfere with circadian rhythms.

Social cues can also affect circadian rhythms. That's why sunshine and communal meals can help travelers overcome jet lag.

Your child's circadian rhythms are partially determined by the environment and partially hard-wired. All people have genes called "clock genes" that determine where they fall on the scale from extreme early bird to extreme night owl.

You might be able to get a night owl to go to bed an hour earlier, but attempts to turn them into a cheerful morning person are doomed to fail. They were born this way. One way you can help your child thrive is to help them learn to understand and work with their natural rhythms. An extreme early bird might be happier doing their homework before school than in the evening. Meanwhile, when a night owl hits high school, she may want to try to schedule her most difficult academic classes for after lunch.

Sleep Changes As People Grow

Sleep patterns do not remain completely consistent over your child's life. They change as your child grows and changes. For instance:

- At birth, your child will spend about 50% of the night in REM sleep. The percentage gradually declines until the child reaches adult levels of 15-20% REM sleep.

- Regular sleep cycles begin to develop around at around 9 weeks old. Initially, each cycle is only about 40 minutes long. By the time a healthy child is a toddler, cycle length has increased to 60 minutes. Finally, around age 5 or 6, cycles reach their adult length – 90 minutes.

- During puberty, teen circadian rhythms shift so that even morning people want to stay up late and then sleep late in the morning. This is one reason that early high school start times are bad for teens.

- As people age, they start going through fewer sleep cycles each night, and their circadian rhythms shift until they are going to be very early and getting up very early.

Why is there so much variation in sleep across the lifespan? Some social biologists think that this variation, and the variation in clock genes, work to ensure that there are always some people awake, working, and keeping watch.

What Do All These Patterns Do For My Child?

These patterns of sleep help your child's brain and body grow, regulate hormones so that your child can let go of stress, control food cravings, and hunger signs, heal injuries, fight disease, and affect how your child learns, thinks, and feels. For our brains and bodies to function correctly, we need to move through all of the sleep stages multiple times a night. When our sleep is interrupted or cut short, we suffer.

Here are just a few fun facts about what different sleep stages do to help your child learn and grow in less obvious ways (Since you already know that deep sleep is necessary for plain old getting taller!)

Sleep empties out the short-term memory so that your child can learn and experience new things. Have you ever felt like your brain was too full and you needed a nap? Kids feel that way too, and the younger the child, the more they're learning and the more they need those naps.

If a kid isn't getting enough sleep or isn't getting the naps they need, the hypothalamus, the part of the brain that stores new information, gets full. They stop being able to learn new things, everything 'falls out of their head,' and they feel overwhelmed and overstimulated.

Sleep spindles in stages 2, 3, and 4 improve learning and long-term memory. Scientists aren't completely sure how these brain waves work, but children with more sleep spindles appear to be better at working around disabilities and memorizing new material. Sleep helps your brain store all that new material where you can access it again later.

Sleep improves muscle memory. Muscle memory is actually "Pattern of movements memory." In the last two hours of an eight-hour stretch of sleep, the brain practices these sequences of signals and movements so that your child can learn to repeat a set of motions without stopping to think.

Children learning new physical skills like swimming or riding a bike lose when they have to get up before their brain is ready. Young drivers learn faster and have fewer accidents if they get more sleep. When athletes don't get enough sleep, they fall more, overextend joints more, and generally injure themselves more. This even affects the elderly. One cause of increased falls may be getting up too early, before the brain has time to consolidate muscle memory.

Sleep also helps us forget unimportant things. Your child needs to remember her math facts or the state capitals. She doesn't need to remember exactly what her best friend was wearing 4 weeks ago. Her brain takes in all this information, but some gets stored and some gets dropped. Sleep is where the brain sorts, catalogs, and stores information so that you can find what you need quickly without distraction.

Sleep helps your child process big emotions and social situations. REM sleep helps us process emotions. Has your child ever had a stressful day and then had a nightmare afterward? That's the brain processing the big emotions and helping your child understand them.

Have you ever had a dream where it seems like your actual interactions with certain people are represented, but in surreal ways? That's also your brain processing complex data. Getting enough sleep helps your learn how to interact, predict other people's actions and reactions, and understand the complex network of social relationships in your life.

Your child needs healthy sleep so that he can navigate the complex feelings and social interactions that fill his day. In fact, researchers are discovering that many children who suffer from ASD also have unusual REM sleep patterns. The inability to navigate social situations and pick up on social cues associated with ASD may be the result of a brain that isn't getting a chance to practice these skills during sleep.

Sleep gives your child the creativity they need to solve problems. REM sleep also recombines everything you know and experience in new and unexpected ways. While some of this helps your child process emotions and social interactions, some of it can help them find new ways to solve difficult problems.

There's a reason that when someone has a problem to solve we suggest that they 'sleep on it.' REM sleep can solve the problem by giving your child new ways to think about it and new solutions to try.

Meet Jackson, The Child Who Gets Enough Sleep

Jackson is ten, and he has no difficulties with sleep. Most days, he wakes up before the alarm clock. He follows his morning routine, eating, bathing, getting dressed, brushing his hair and teeth, and doing a morning chore. He doesn't lose his shoes, and he doesn't need to rush. He can focus and get out the door on time.

At school, Jackson is a pretty good kid. He's not the teacher's pet, but he's not a troublemaker. He does fine in classes and has clear strengths and weaknesses. He gets along well with the other children. He can sit quietly in class, is a voracious eater at lunch, and enjoys getting exercise at recess.

He enjoys his after-school activities and his coaches like him. After a long day and a good dinner, his mom has to remind him to do his homework, but he finishes quickly. He can navigate his bedtime routine and goes to bed tired but not exhausted.

Jackson still has his moments. Sometimes he fights with his sister, talks back, or ignores his teachers, but he's a happy, healthy, well-adjusted kid as long as he sleeps well, eats healthy, and gets enough exercise every day.

CHANGE THE SLEEP, CHANGE THE CHILD'S LIFE

What would your child look like as a Jackson? Would she finally have the attention and focus to excel at the sport she loves? Would he be able to learn new skills and enjoy gardening and woodworking? Would school stop being torture, would life stop being so hard, would your child be able to just enjoy being a kid without so many struggles?

If sleep is the cause of your child's difficulties, your child can have this kind of unburdened life. When we change the sleep and cure the sleep problems, we give a child's brain and body the chance to grow, thrive, and be happy.

In the next chapter, you'll learn about some of the most common reasons that our kids aren't getting sleep, and which specialists can help your children get diagnosed and treated.

CHAPTER 3
SLEEP THIEVES

By now, you're probably convinced that your child is living in a constant state of sleep deprivation. And you know what? You're most likely right. According to the National Sleep Foundation, 52% of K-8 children and 87% of teens are not getting enough sleep at night.

If your child is not acting like a healthy, well-rested youth, it is extremely likely that the underlying cause is a lack of good healthy sleep, either going to sleep too late, getting up too early, or both. It's time to learn about the sneaky thieves who are stealing your child's sleep.

Modern Living is Anti-Sleep

As an adult trying to balance work, family, and a tiny sliver of time for yourself, you probably let sleep slip sometimes, even though you know how much you need it. Your kids have less developed brains and so are even worse at navigating sleep and life than you are. How are your kids doing in these areas?

Bedtime is not for screen time.

The blue light from screens (or certain fluorescent and LED bulbs) can mess with your circadian rhythms. Why? Because your eyes play an important role in regulating your sleep-wake schedule. This is why the advice for an infant who has "days and nights mixed up" is time out in the sunshine.

Remember, our brains are designed for a time before screens, or even light bulbs. The warmer, orangish light of late afternoon and early evening triggers a hormone release that says "Time to wind down for bed!"

Meanwhile, the harsh, blue light of screens and certain bulbs sends the opposite message. "Wake up! There is a lot of stuff to do!"

For kids (and adults) this quickly becomes a sleep-stealing feedback loop. It's late, but your kid is on a screen, so she isn't sleepy. She's not sleepy, so she leaves the screen on. Before long, it's after midnight, she's exhausted, and she just missed out on the part of her night devoted to healing, restorative sleep and remembering what she learned in school.

How to fix the problem

Experts recommend ditching the screens about 2 hours before bedtime, but for the best sleep, go a step further.

Ditch the TV and screens after supper, and go outside for a family walk, or just relax on the patio. Let your brain get a look at some of that evening sunshine, and reset yourself for a good night's sleep.

Alternatively, there are now smart lightbulbs that change the color and intensity of household light to support healthy circadian rhythms. These can help if you're looking to have a "smart home," but if you just want to be conscious of how light affects your child's brain, try the walk!

School schedules make it hard to respect sleep needs

When your child was small, you may have been able to get them to bed by 7 so they had a good night's sleep before school. Now, they're a teen, and suddenly everything has changed. They want to stay up later than you do, but they have to be up at the crack of dawn for school. They say they're just not sleepy at 9 pm, but you can see them sleepwalking through their days.

Sound familiar? That's because teen brains naturally shift bedtimes and waking times later. It's part of growing up, but it's also a big problem for American teens today. Why? Because school systems don't respect teen schedule needs.

Our teens are waking up too early, so they miss out on some of their REM sleep, the phase of sleep most necessary for navigating complex emotional and social situations, right at the time when their whole life is one big complex emotional and social situation!

It gets worse. It means that our kids aren't fully awake for their morning classes, so that first-period math is a disaster. Then, you have these kids driving to and from school and activities while they're chronically exhausted. The lack of good sleep slows their reaction times and is a big contributor to why teen drivers are exhausted drivers.

Our schedules are not supporting our children's sleep needs, and it has a huge impact on your teen's health and learning.

How to fix the problem

First of all, be understanding. It's not that your kid is rebelling against bedtimes, it's that their brain is telling them to stay up later and to sleep in. This is a normal part of the massive changes that happen in an adolescent brain. (You may see the flip side of this in your aging parents or relatives. Are they suddenly going to bed before you've had dinner? The elderly often experience a circadian rhythm shift where they go to bed and get up much earlier.)

Secondly, advocate for later high school start times in your district. In a study from the University of Kentucky, researchers found that later high school start times increased achievement and reduced the number of teen car accidents. Teen sleep isn't just about moods and test scores, it's a matter of life and death.

Finally, if your teen must attend school early, have them try to schedule their hardest classes later in the day, not earlier. If possible, avoid having them drive to and from school, since drowsy driving can cause accidents. If they must drive, remind them that reaching a destination safely is always more important than getting there on time.

Exercise enhances sleep

Have you ever been sick, too tired to get out of bed, and yet not at all sleepy? It's a horrible feeling, isn't it? Many children have that feeling every night at bedtime. They just can't sleep, and one piece of the puzzle is exercise.

Think back to your own childhood. You probably ran for hours after school and played outside all day in the summer. Your school days were shorter, and they had more recesses and more "special" time built into them.

Our children don't have that kind of freedom to run off their energy. School and play are more sedentary than they were 20-30 years ago, and it is hurting our kids. Their sleep is disrupted because they aren't getting enough physical activity during the day.

How to fix the problem

If your kid is athletic, they're probably on teams that make sure they train and get exercise. But what about less athletic kids in areas where rec leagues die out by third or fourth grade?

This is where being active as a family comes in. Remember that after-dinner family walk that I mentioned? It's not just great for the brain, it's great for the body! If you have access to a park or a yard, go out and play frisbee or soccer with your kids. You don't have to be good at a sport to connect, have fun, and be together in the great outdoors.

On weekends, start taking family hikes or bike rides. If you live in a walkable area, encourage your child to walk along with you on errands. Getting out and getting moving makes it easier to sleep at night and will support everyone's health and growth.

Some Kids Are Born Bad Sleepers

Did you know that when you wake and when you sleep isn't just about willpower? In addition to the circadian rhythm shifts as a result of growing and aging, some parts of your sleep cycle are encoded into your very DNA. This is why some families have babies who sleep through the night on day one, and other families have three-year-olds who are perfectly healthy but can't sleep before midnight.

Wondering why your kids are such terrible sleepers? Ask both sets of grandparents about their experiences with babies and sleep. But watch out, they may just laugh and say that you've been blessed with children who are just like you and your spouse.

Here are a few of the most common ways that genes can affect your child's sleep.

Tick Tock, Tick Tock, there's a clock inside your genes.

Every human has a section of DNA devoted to clock genes. These genes determine when you'll get sleepy at night and when you'll wake up. However, there are many different ways these genes can work.

Some people naturally go to bed very early and wake up very early. These people do great as farmers, or as people who work the 7-3 shift. Other people are natural 'night people.' They are wakeful at night and sleepy during the day – and it's good we have them! We need our night workers like police, nurses, overnight IT workers, and night shift security and cleaning teams! Most of us fall somewhere in the middle.

Scientists think we have this huge range of sleeping times because all human societies, from hunter-gatherers to modern America, need some people awake at all times of day. Clock genes mean that instead of having the person who turns into a pumpkin at 10 pm working overnight in the ER, we can have a doctor who is alert, awake, and at their best. They're a blessing.

Well, they're a blessing to adults. For kids whose preferred sleeping times are outside the norm, clock genes can be a curse, because, unlike adults, kids can't choose when to live the "productive time" of day. They're tied down to the school and activity schedules that are based around the "typical" child and parent needs.

Do you have a toddler who wants to sleep from midnight to 11 am? It's not your parenting. Look at your family tree. Chances are, you have some family members who thrived on night shifts. Do you have a kid who crashes right after dinner, but is up and alert at 4 am? Looks like you've given birth to the second coming of Uncle Pete, the successful dairy farmer.

What to do about it

You can't totally change your child's clock genes, but you can nudge them a little and try to make life a bit easier for them.

- If your kid is a night owl, try taking the advice on good bedtime behaviors, and you might be able to nudge sleep a little later. By helping your child feel tired earlier and wind down faster, you might shave an hour or so off their bedtime.

- Help your child be aware of their tendencies, and give them coping tools to help them shift their hardest thinking to times of day when they're awake.

- For instance, a kid who crashes at 6 pm but wakes at 4 am might be happier doing hard homework assignments in the morning, when their brain works. As they get older, these quiet hours might be a great time for meal prep and batch cooking, so they don't have to think about food when they're exhausted.

- On weekends, summers, and vacations, let your kid respect their internal clock. These are great times for your kids to learn how their bodies work when they're not forced onto a schedule made for someone else. They can learn to love their quirky clocks and develop their own strategies for coping.

- Help them see how their clock genes are ultimately a strength. This is especially important for those night owls. As a society, we often glorify people who keep 'farmer hours' as hardworking go-getters, and call our night owls "lazybones." (On the flip side, when those natural farmers hit their young adult years, their early bedtimes can hold them back socially and leave them open to mockery.) So help your child love their genes. Their personal sleep patterns should not affect their self-esteem.

Is your child a mutant?

Mutations to key genes can also cause your child to have sleep issues. Some children (and adults) simply cannot make and process

Melatonin correctly. Melatonin is a hormone that helps regulate your sleep and your body and brain's actions during sleep.

If you don't have enough melatonin, you won't feel sleepy, even when your body is exhausted. You also won't have the ability to stay asleep. People who lack melatonin often can only complete about half a night's sleep.

What to do about it

If you suspect a melatonin deficiency, talk to your pediatrician about next steps.

There are tests that can help you determine if a mutation is at the root of your family's sleep issues. If your child doesn't have the mutation, melatonin supplements won't do them much good on the sleep front, so it's worth investigating before you try to supplement.

Non-Neurotypical kids often have non-neurotypical sleep patterns

Sometimes, a kid with poor sleep is diagnosed with Attention Deficit Hyperactive Disorder (ADHD) or Autism Spectrum Disorder (ASD) because the lack of sleep causes behaviors that mimic these conditions. However, researchers have found that children who have these conditions also have underlying sleep difficulties.

These conditions, and sleep and brain differences, are increasingly detectable in early infancy, and that's one reason why the mothers of kids with these disorders are so tired. Their kids just don't have brains that are wired for sleep.

What to do about it

There are sleep clinics and psychologists who specialize in helping ADHD and ASD kids get to sleep, but the wait lists are very long. In the meantime, get your child checked for other underlying conditions that could be making their sleep issues even worse. Know that your kid isn't a bad kid. They're not doing this on purpose, their brains are keeping them up.

Do your best to promote exercise, a healthy diet, and a good night's sleep, but know when to throw in the towel. Find ways to get some respite so that you, at least, can sleep, even if your child cannot. Keep up on the current research about kids like yours and sleep, and do your best. It's an exhausting situation, but as they age, many non-neurotypical kids improve their sleep skills.

WHAT YOUR KID EATS CAN CHANGE HOW THEY SLEEP

We've talked about how exercise and screen time can affect your kids' sleep. Did you know that nutrition also plays an important role in getting to bed and sleeping through the night?

That's one reason babies, and especially breastfed babies, sleep in smaller stretches. When your body needs nutrition, it wakes up! For a baby, a small stomach and easily digestible food are the culprits, and the frequent waking helps them grow and learn.

For older children, a healthy diet should provide all the nutrition they need to sleep through the night. If your child isn't sleeping it's time to look at the timing and content of their meals.

Vitamins support great sleep

What you eat affects how you sleep. If your child is a picky eater, their diet could be affecting their sleep. Here are some of the vitamins and minerals they need to sleep, and where to find them in a healthy diet.

Stop the twitch with adequate iron

Restless leg syndrome can keep a child from falling or staying asleep. Kids with RLS literally hurt if they stay still. Every fiber of their being is causing them to thrash around, either just before or just after they sleep.

A common cause of RLS is iron deficiency. If your child appears to suffer from twitchy legs at bedtime, ask your pediatrician to check their ferritin levels. Making sure that they have enough iron in their diet or, if necessary, iron supplements can help support healthy sleep.

For better sleep, get vitamin D

Many children, especially those in northern latitudes, just don't get enough vitamin D in the winter. Our bodies can make their own vitamin D when we get sunshine, but when it's cold and dark, and kids spend all their daylight hours in the classroom, their health, and their sleep, suffers.

In the US, milk products are fortified with vitamin D, but what do you do for a child who doesn't like or can't tolerate milk? Supplements are one answer, of course, but you can also introduce vitamin D into the diet by adding egg yolks or salmon to your child's meal rotation.

Vitamins C and E promote healthy rest

Vitamins C and E don't just promote your immune system. They also help you breathe better in your sleep.

Your child can get enough of these vitamins by eating plenty of fruit, nuts, and leafy greens. If you have a picky eater, you may need to look into a supplement, but as always, vitamins work best when your child gets them by eating a varied diet full of natural, whole foods!

Vitamin B6 aids in melatonin production

A B6 deficiency can affect your child's ability to make and use melatonin.

Get your child plenty of B6 with foods like leafy greens, chickpeas, fish, and poultry. Or, if you have a picky eater, fortified breakfast cereals can provide a decent source of this nutrient.

B12 is essential for circadian rhythms

Vitamin B12 regulates your child's circadian rhythms and is essential for health. The bad news is that this vitamin is only found in animal products.

Meat and fish contain enough B12 to support human health, but vegetarians are also safe. Dairy products like milk, yogurt and cheese, and even eggs are good sources of this essential nutrient.

If your family is vegan or your child is a very picky eater, it can be nearly impossible to get sufficient B12 through your diet. If you suspect your child may not be getting enough of this essential nutrient to support sleep and growth, talk to your pediatrician and have their levels tested.

Stop midnight munchies with the right kind of bedtime snacks

Many kids get sweets as a last treat before bed. If you want your child to sleep well, move the sweet treat to earlier in the night, and make sure that the bedtime snack has a good balance of protein, whole grains, and fat that will stick with your child all night and support healthy rest and healing. Some great snacks to help younger kids sleep better include:

- An egg scrambled with cheese on whole wheat toast
- Hummus and veggies
- Plain Greek yogurt and fruit
- A peanut butter and jelly sandwich
- Oatmeal made with milk and nuts
- Fruit and cottage cheese

The snack should not be as big as a regular meal, but it should be nourishing enough to get them through the work of sleep and to let them wake up happy.

Warm milk or herbal tea can help a child wind down

Sometimes, a child is well-nourished and not hungry but still needs to relax and wind down. Warm milk or a sleep-promoting herbal tea like chamomile can help them relax and feel sleepy.

SOMETIMES, THE INABILITY TO SLEEP IS ALL IN THEIR MIND

Have you ever been really worried about work or finances, and then found that you can't sleep at night? You might lie awake in bed ruminating, chewing over your problems just like a cow chews its cud for hours and hours until finally, the sun rises and you give up on sleep and resign yourself to an awful day.

Children also experience sleep issues due to anxieties, but they don't always know how to explain their worries to their parents. They often tell parents that they're not tired, that they're thinking too hard, or that they have had or are afraid they will have nightmares. Anxiety that disrupts sleep can be a normal developmental phase or a sign of a larger problem.

To help your children overcome anxiety before sleep, make the bedroom a calm place. Their bed should only be used for sleeping or for reading before bed. Before bed, practice calming breathing or gentle yoga routines. Read a soothing story and play calm music or white noise.

If helping your children wind their minds down before sleep doesn't help, it may be time to talk to your pediatrician to rule out underlying causes and to find expert help for dealing with anxiety in children and teens.

Illnesses, Allergies, and Asthma

If children are stuffy and cannot breathe, they cannot sleep. This is why allergic kids often have "raccoon eyes," big purple circles around their eyes. Kids with nasal congestion, coughing, and wheezing aren't sleeping.

When your child has a fleeting illness, you can try to make them comfortable and hope that they recover quickly. But for kids with allergies, especially dust, pollen, and mold allergies, or with asthma, you need to take more drastic steps to assure them a good night's sleep.

- **Remember that asthma isn't just wheezing.** Does your kid have a nagging cough on and off all night that never seems to wake them? That cab be a sign of asthma. See your pediatrician immediately so you can keep the lungs from getting more damaged and the asthma from getting worse.

- **Allergen-proof the sleeping area.** Allergic and asthmatic kids are more vulnerable at night because they're spending 8 hours breathing in the same allergens over and over. To reduce allergies:
    - Invest in a good HEPA filter to clean the air while they sleep
    - Enclose sheets and pillows in hypoallergenic dust covers
    - If possible, replace carpet with wood or laminate flooring
    - Get that dirty laundry off the floor, into a hamper, and out of the room. (This can be extra hard with teens.)
    - Wash all bedding once a week on hot, regardless of what the label says. (This may shorten the life of the fabric, but it extends the life of your kids' lungs.)
    - Limit stuffies on the bed, and if possible keep them off the bed altogether.

These changes can be hard to make, but they'll help your child get the sleep they need by controlling asthma and allergies.

When the Airway is Blocked

Most of the sleep thieves you've met so far are pretty easy to defeat. You, as a parent, can help your children navigate many of these struggles so that they can get better sleep and live happier, healthier lives.

When a child's airway is restricted or blocked during sleep, they struggle to breathe. They wake up to gasp for breath or change position, but only for a few seconds. In the morning they won't remember these microarousals, but over the course of a night they have a huge impact on your child's sleep.

Think about the work of healing, growth, and memory that happens during deep sleep. For your child's body and brain to grow, they need long periods of deep sleep.

When the airway is blocked, the child only gets a few seconds or minutes of healing deep sleep at a time. Their body can't release hormones properly. They don't grow taller, they don't remember what they learn in school, their bodies can't heal. They never feel rested in the morning because they never got real sleep. They're sick, but no blood test can diagnose what's wrong.

There are two main kinds of airway issues that are common in children in teens: UARS and OSA.

UARS can be easy to overlook

In Upper Airway Resistance Syndrome (UARS), the airway isn't completely blocked, but it is partially closed. As a result, the child struggles to breathe and must change position frequently to catch their breath.

Often, these children have severe allergies or some sort of palate or sinus malformation which means that there is less room in their sinus cavities to begin with. In children, the most common cause of this is a high and narrow hard palate. The hard palate is the floor of the sinus cavity. When it's high and narrow it constricts the cavity and makes it harder for air to move through the sinuses. This means that, even under the best of circumstances, that child is struggling to breathe normally while they sleep.

Small setbacks like a cold or allergy season can totally block the sinuses and nose, turning the child into a mouth breather. This starts a cycle of issues that can eventually progress to full-blown obstructive sleep apnea, or OSA. In the next chapter, we'll take a closer look at why UARS is so serious.

OSA: What is blocking my child's airway?

Obstructive sleep apnea occurs when the airway becomes totally blocked during sleep. These kids aren't just struggling to breathe well. They can't breathe at all. Every night they experience multiple periods where they stop breathing and their brains are deprived of oxygen.

OSA symptoms are usually far more severe than UARS symptoms because a simple change of position won't help these kids. They have to wake up and gasp for air, and their obstruction makes breathing impossible even when they're not sick or having an allergy flare.

So, what's blocking the airway in these kids? OSA in children is often a combination of a few different factors.

1. Habitual mouth-breathers suck in dry air, unfiltered air. Usually, the nose and sinuses filter, warm, and humidify your breath so that it doesn't irritate your airway and lungs. Mouth breathers bypass this important system.

2. This air irritates the tonsils and adenoids and causes them to swell, reducing the space in the airway.

3. If a child has an overbite, their jaw and tongue move backward during sleep as well.

4. The tongue flops back in the throat, covers the windpipe, and completes the obstructive process.

5. Children with unreleased tongue ties experience a similar phenomenon even if they don't have an overbite. This is because their tongues rest in the middle or bottom of

their mouths instead of the palate, so during sleep, they flop back and obstruct the airway.

What to do about it

When a child has UARS or OSA, they need to be screened and treated by a trained professional who can open the airway. When the underlying structural problems that cause mouth breathing or obstructions from the tongue are treated, children learn to breathe normally. They start sleeping and getting real, restorative sleep. Finally, they're able to live normal lives and enjoy their childhoods.

Further reading for Chapter 3
https://www.ncbi.nlm.nih.gov/pmc/articles/PMC2603528/

CHAPTER 4
AIRWAY UP CLOSE

Now that you understand how important sleep is to your child, and what can steal sleep away, it's time to take a closer look at the airway. When your airway is working well, you hardly know it's there at all. You notice it when you're having trouble breathing or when your nose and sinuses get clogged. However, the airway is an essential part of your body.

Every cell in our body needs oxygen to function. Without oxygen, cells can't make the energy they need to function and grow. That's why when someone has bronchitis or pneumonia, they feel fuzzy-brained and exhausted. A clogged, blocked, or irritated airway means less air. Less air means less oxygen, and less oxygen means the body starts falling apart. This is why I like to tell the parents of my patients that "Airway is life."

THE UPPER AIRWAY AND ITS ROLE DURING SLEEP

To understand what happens when airways go wrong, it helps to know what they look like when everything is going right. Your airway is every place that air passes through on its journey from your mouth and nose to your lungs.

Doctors divide the airway into two parts, the upper airway, and the lower airway. Your larynx, or voice box, is the dividing line between the two and can be considered the end of the upper or the beginning of the lower, depending on your doctor. Your lower airway is your trachea, bronchial tubes (the part that gets tight and hurts when someone has bronchitis or an asthma attack), and your lungs, which transfer oxygen from the air to your blood, and carbon dioxide from your blood to the air.

The upper airway is the part of the airway that is affected by UARS and OSA. It includes your nose, sinuses, mouth, and pharynx, the part of the throat that food travels through on its way to the esophagus and stomach, and that air travels through on its way to the lower airway.

WHAT GOOD ARE NOSES AND SINUSES?

Your nose and sinus aren't just the easiest way to breathe, they're the best way to breathe! That's because these structures are designed to protect your bronchiole tubes and lungs from damage.

Think about all the places that you breathe over the course of your life. Sometimes, the air is hot, sometimes it's freezing cold. Sometimes it's too humid and sometimes it's too dry. Air can be full of dust, mold and pollen, and it can be full of bacteria and viruses. You'd have to be crazy to just let it straight into your lungs!

And that's why healthy people breathe all that unpredictable air in through their noses.

As air travels through your nose and sinuses, a few important things happen to it.

The nose and sinuses control the temperature of the air. As the air passes through your nose and sinuses, it becomes closer to body temperature. Hot air cools down and cold air warms up to protect your lungs.

The nose and sinuses control the humidity of the air. This journey also adjusts the humidity of the air, especially dry air, so that it is less likely to irritate your throat and lungs.

The nose and sinuses filter out irritants. Everyone's nose has nose hairs growing inside of it. These hairs are coated in a sticky mucus. When you breathe in particles of pollen or dust, the hairs trap it to keep it out of your lungs. If the air is too dusty or it's the height of pollen season, some of the detritus still gets through, but your nose hair still does a great job keeping the dust and pollen out of your lungs until you're ready to sneeze it out!

The nose and sinuses fight bacteria and viruses. We tend to think of mucus in our nose and sinuses as a bad thing. After all, it's caused by illnesses, right? Well, not exactly. Viruses and bacteria don't produce mucus. Our body makes mucus to fight bacteria and viruses. The mucus traps the germs and allows our immune systems to identify and trap them. By providing this barrier, our nose and sinuses keep diseases from reaching our bronchiole tubes and lungs, where they'd much more serious than just a nasty, snotty cold.

Once the air has traveled through your sinuses, it heads down your throat, or pharynx. Your throat also has mucus that can trap particles and germs, and your tonsils and adenoids can release immune cells that fight disease.

Now we come to a fork in the road..er.. airway. Air leaving your pharynx can go one of two ways. Into your lower airway, or down your esophagus and into your stomach, where it can cause painful gas. What keeps the air on the right track? Your tongue!

Your tongue controls the exits of the pharynx. When you're breathing, it covers the esophagus so all of the air goes down the larynx. When you're eating, it covers the larynx so that food and liquid go down the esophagus and you don't aspirate them into your lungs. When it can do its job well, the tongue is an important part of your airway.

Ok, but what about the mouth?

Your mouth also plays an important role in the upper airway.

Your mouth is your backup breather. The nose is great, but it takes air in slowly. When you need a burst of air quickly, like if you've just had a heavy workout, you instinctively begin to breathe through your mouth. This air isn't as good for your lungs, but you can get a lot of it fast.

Your mouth also kicks in when your nose and sinuses are obstructed and can't move air easily. This is why kids with untreated allergies are often mouth-breathers.

The roof of your mouth is the bottom of your sinus cavity. Feel the roof of your mouth with your tongue. That's your hard palate. Your hard palate is the floor of your sinus cavity. It grows and changes throughout childhood, and affects the shape of your face and whether you have room for your adult teeth. If it's too high and narrow, it can reduce the capacity of your sinuses and make it harder to breathe, especially when you have allergies or a cold.

Your mouth helps control the airflow out of your body. Have you ever tried to blow out a candle with your nose? It won't work! But we can blow out candles without mouths. Our lips, cheeks, tongue, and teeth all work together to help us direct and change the shape of the air we exhale. This helps us sing, speak, and blow up balloons. When these parts can't work together well, it impacts our breathing.

Your tongue helps keep the airway open at night. We already talked about how the tongue acts as a traffic controller between the airway and the esophagus. It also has a role to play in sleep breathing. Healthy sleepers rest their tongue on the roof of their mouths during sleep. This keeps their airways clear and helps breathing. When the tongue rests lower in the mouth and you lay on your back, it will block your larynx and cause sleep breathing problems.

How Do Kids Get UARS or OSA?

We usually think of Obstructive Sleep Apnea or Upper Airway Resistance Syndrome as things that affect older, obese people. So how can a tiny child have the same issues that her grandfather does?

There are a few key points to remember:

- While obesity can make OSA and UARS worse, often the disease precedes, and causes, weight gain. We're not catching this illness until years of dysregulated hormones have led to weight gain, but when we treat it earlier, we can prevent the obesity.

- Many children have congenital traits that make OSA more likely. Sometimes, OSA is in the cards before they're born.

- OSA and UARS are treatable, even in kids! When we identify and treat a child who has sleep breathing issues, we address the root causes. We're not just making them healthier now, we're helping them stay healthier for the rest of their lives.

- The most obvious thing blocking the airway is not always the underlying cause of OSA. That means simply removing the blockage may provide immediate relief, but still leaves your child at risk for developing adult OSA later in life.

What is blocking my child's airway?

If a pediatrician has screened your child for sleep problems, they may have checked your child's tonsils and adenoids for swelling. That's because, in many children with OSA, these glands are inflamed and have grown to fully or partially block the airway during sleep. In fact, often the first line of treatment is to remove the tonsils and adenoids on the grounds that they are an obvious source of blockage.

However, this approach often ignores the fact that tonsils and adenoids don't swell without reason. They swell because they are fighting diseases or because they've become irritated for some reason. These swollen glands are often the most obvious symptom of a larger problem.

How Tonsils and Adenoids can Swell

Connie is a mouth breather. She breathes through her mouth at school and when she watches TV. It's almost as if, during the day, she doesn't know that her nose exists. At night, she snores, chokes and gags. When she goes to the pediatrician, her tonsils and adenoids are swollen. This must be the cause of her problems! She has them removed, and her night breathing improves, but she still breathes mostly through her mouth.

Engineers use a system called "5 Whys" to find the root cause of a problem. Look how Connie's story changes when we use the 5 whys!

1. Connie's Tonsils and Adenoids are swollen. Why?

2. They are irritated and constantly fighting pathogens. Why?

3. Connie breathes through her mouth, so the nose and sinuses aren't doing their job. Why?

4. Connie's nose and sinuses are just too hard to breathe through. Why?

5. Connie has a high narrow palate, so air can't move through her nasal cavity easily.

Using the 5 Whys method in this case might leave you with one final question. "Why is Connie's palate high and narrow?"

For kids who don't have an obvious genetic syndrome, the answer is often "tongue and lip ties."

How Tongue Tie impacts the development of the airway, and other parts of life too!

Tongue tie is a condition where bands of tissue tether the tongue to the floor of your mouth. A normal tongue can move freely. A tied tongue can't reach the roof of the mouth, has trouble shaping the air for speech, and has a harder time moving food around the mouth when you're eating. It adds up to big problems, especially for sleep breathing.

How do kids get tongue tie?

Tongue tie is something that happens during fetal development. If a child is tongue-tied, they were tongue-tied in the womb. Tongue-tie is what is called a midline deformity, and it sometimes it clusters with other issues, like heart defects or bladder problems.

It can occur because of:

- **Genetic predisposition.** It runs in families. Often adults discover their history of tongue tie-related health issues when their children are diagnosed.

- **Environmental toxins or viral exposure during pregnancy.** Toxins in the environment and certain viruses seem to be linked to tongue -tie and other fetal abnormalities. But it's a complicated mix where some children are already genetically predisposed, and others are not.

- **Folic Acid deficiencies during pregnancy.** If you took your prenatal vitamins religiously, you may wonder how your child could be suffering from the results of a folic acid deficiency. Increasingly, the answer appears to be "an MTHFR mutation." This gene influences how the body processes folic acid.

- ○ People with certain gene variations can't process the artificial form of folic acid found in fortified foods and most vitamins. When mom, baby, or both has this mutation, there is a higher rate of midline deformities. (In fact, variations to this gene may explain some of the 'runs in the family' aspect of tongue ties.)

Your child's tongue tie is not your fault, and is fixable, especially if we catch it before they are an adult.

HOW DOES TONGUE TIE AFFECT GROWTH AND DEVELOPMENT?

Palate formation. Tongue tie doesn't just affect the tongue. From before a child is born, it affects their palate and facial development. Normally, the tongue acts as a natural retainer and palate spreader. Even before birth, when it rests in the roof of the mouth it helps the palate become wide and flat. This gives the child a bigger sinus cavity and more room for their baby and adult teeth.

When the tongue is tied, it can't perform its job in palate formation. The palate remains high and narrow. The child has sinuses that won't function well, and an upper jaw that won't have room for all of their adult teeth. That means expensive orthodontics down the line, and nasal breathing problems and sleep breathing problems their entire life.

Feeding Difficulties

Infants with tongue ties can be difficult to nurse. To get milk from the breast, babies use their tongues while they suck. If the tongue doesn't have the full range of motion, the child can't efficiently drain the breast.

This means you end up with:

- A baby who nurses 24-7 and seldom stops for more than a few minutes at a time

- Slow growth and lack of chubbiness despite all the time spent nursing

- Poor sleep – they can't sleep two hours straight, because they need that time to eat

- Constant crying and hysteria if removed from the breast – these kids are genuinely hungry

- Painful nursing for mom. Without the help of the tongue, they're using suction alone.

- Nipples deformed after nursing – they look like fresh tubes of lipstick

- Cracked and bleeding nipples – Breasts aren't designed to take this kind of abuse!

- Mastitis because the baby isn't fully draining the breasts with each feed

For some babies, even bottles are too difficult to use. Fortunately, these kids tend to lose weight so rapidly that they get treatment for their ties by the time they're a week or two old.

Eventually, most of these poor nursers grow up, but only after a lot of mental and physical anguish for mom and baby. So what happens when they start on solids and cups? More trouble.

Your tongue works hard when you eat and drink. When you drink, it has to cover the larynx and help you swallow liquid. When you eat, it moves food around the mouth to help you chew and mash it, and to help keep it from getting stuck in your palate or teeth. Then it helps you swallow while also covering the larynx to prevent aspiration.

So, when a mildly tongue-tied kid moves to food, what you get is a **CHOKEY** kid. These kids always seem to gag, choke, and end up with 'too much food to chew.' It's not deliberate and it's not eating too fast. It's that an essential part of their mouth isn't working right. These kids often become "fussy eaters," especially when it comes to texture. Basically, they've learned what foods they can't chew and swallow well, so they avoid them.

Speech difficulties

So many of our consonant sounds need the tongue to be able to reach the roof of the mouth! And even vowels need the tongue to help shape the sounds so that the difference in vowel sounds is clear. A kid who has a tongue tie will have a harder time learning to make normal speech sounds. They'll often need speech therapy, and won't be able to truly master Ls and Rs until their tie is revised.

Sleep breathing difficulties

Tongue-tied kids snore more because their tongue is partially obstructing the airway during sleep. Since they can't raise it and rest it in the roof of the mouth, it flops backward and causes problems. This leads to bedwetting, interrupted sleep, and ultimately poor growth, poor health, and poor academic performance because the brain and body aren't doing the work of sleep.

Why tongue ties don't get treated in infancy

With so many negative effects from tongue ties, you're probably wondering why tongue ties aren't revised immediately. When the tethered tongue of a newborn is released, it's literally a 90-second procedure and a single drop of blood. The most traumatic part for the baby is that for about 30 of those 90 seconds adults hold their hands and heads still.

As soon as the tongue tie is released, the baby can nurse vigorously. They have years for their tongue to widen their palates. They learn to speak normally, and they breathe well while they sleep. Moms who have experienced the change often describe it as "like a whole different child" because their clingy baby who is only happy when nursing becomes a full, content, cheerful, easygoing child.

Until the mid-20th century, it was the standard of care to release all ties at birth so that kids could eat and grow well. Before the invention of baby formula, tongue tie was literally a matter of life or death. However, once most families began using formula and bottles, the practice of releasing all ties immediately fell out of use.

Now, many pediatricians will not release a tie unless a child is dropping off the growth chart, regardless of how much pain the tie causes mom and baby. The logic is that the procedure is unnecessary because many ties will eventually loosen or break on their own.

However, this is "Pediatrician" logic, not dentist, occupational therapist, or speech pathology logic.

Imagine that the tie breaks on its own at age 6. This child has already missed out on 6 years of palate development and is looking at a long future of orthodontic work to spread the palate and realign the teeth.

The child has missed out on 6 years where new foods can be an adventure, and instead has a limited set of favorite foods. They'll need occupational therapy to learn to eat and swallow properly, and to learn to try and enjoy new foods.

The child has spent 6 years unable to make normal sounds and learning bad habits to cope with their uncooperative tongue. They'll need years of speech and language pathology to correct the problem.

Pediatricians can have tunnel vision because their appointments are mainly focused on "is the child still on the growth chart?" They don't see the effects of an unreleased tie because other specialties treat those effects. And, while we love to get to know your children and help them live healthy lives, we'd rather they be healthy from the start and never need our specialty care.

While it's easiest to release tongue ties in infancy, even adults with tongue ties can benefit from the surgery to sever the tissue and release the tongue. If you suspect that your children, or that you, have an unreleased tongue tie, get help. It could make a huge difference in your life and health.

CHAPTER 5

RESTORE SLEEP, SAVE THE CHILD

Now that you understand how to spot the signs of a sleep problem in your child, you probably have one big question: *How can I get this treated and help my child live a happy, healthy life?* This chapter is everything you need to get your child screened and treated: Who to ask for help, what tests your child will need, and what treatment options are available to get your kids the help they need to breathe better and sleep better.

I'M WORRIED ABOUT MY KID. WHO CAN I TALK TO?

It depends on where you live. Unfortunately, many parts of our country are underserved when it comes to pediatric sleep difficulties, and connecting with the right provider can take time. Here are a few places to start.

Your Child's Dentist

Did you know that dentists are quickly becoming the easiest-to-access pediatric sleep medicine providers? If you express your concerns to your dentist, your child can get a thorough examination of the mouth, tongue, palate, and throat. If your dentist hasn't trained in sleep apnea, palates, and tongue ties yet, don't give up. You might have to drive, but if you suspect that a tongue tie or palate issue is contributing to your child's sleep issues, you'll want to consult with an expert who understands pediatric mouths.

Your Pediatrician or Family Practice Doctor

Your pediatrician may be able to recommend good specialists in your area to investigate sleep issues. A word of warning, however – pediatricians are generalists. This means they may not have the experience or equipment to examine your child for obstructions during a normal appointment.

If you think something is wrong, push for a referral. Most children are never screened for snoring or sleep issues by their primary care provider, even though the American Academy of Pediatrics has recommended annual screenings since 2012. ***Don't be afraid to be that 'pushy' mom who advocates for her child.***

The Family Allergist

If anyone in your family already sees an allergist, this can be a good place to start. Your allergist can determine if sleep breathing problems and mouth breathing are being exacerbated by allergies and asthma. Since these conditions often run in families, it might help to start with someone who is familiar with your family's allergy history.

An Ear, Nose, and Throat Specialist

If your child already has an ear, nose, and throat (ENT) specialist, this can be a good place to start. ENTs tend to focus on the tonsils and adenoids, however, so be sure to ask about being evaluated for other structural issues.

Your Child's Speech and Language Pathologist or Occupational Therapist

Many of the kids I see in my practice already have an OT or SLP in their lives. The same structures that affect their sleep breathing cause other issues that need intervention, or the lack of sleep itself has caused developmental delays. These therapists often have many patients with pediatric OSA, and they can point you to the practitioners in the region who will evaluate and treat kids just like yours.

Other Moms

When all else fails, ask other moms, either in person or in online groups. You are not alone, and you may be surprised how many people can point you to physicians, specialists, and dentists who will take your concerns seriously and give your child a thorough examination. Many of the moms in my practice found me because they asked other moms for advice. Don't be shy about asking for help and advice. The goal is to get your child seen and treated so that she can finally live her life.

What Will My Child's Diagnostic Process for OSA Look Like?

When a practitioner suspects a child might have OSA, we go through several steps to ensure that every kid gets the right diagnosis and the treatment that's right for them. This process can include:

- Screening
- Comprehensive Examination
- Referral to another specialist
- Sleep study
- Treatment options ranging from medication and therapy to surgery, orthodontics, or medical devices.

The exact journey is different for every kid and varies depending on severity, genetics, and age. Let's look at each step in depth so that you can get an idea of what to expect as you begin this process with your child.

Screening

Screening for pediatric sleep apnea begins with questionnaires. These let the practitioner understand what symptoms your child currently exhibits and how they affect daily life for your child and the people around him.

IMPORTANT: ***Do not minimize*** on the questionnaires as they are what opens the door to diagnosis and treatment. Don't picture your child on his best day as you answer – answer based on his worst days. Our goal is to get to the point where his worst days are no worse than any other kid's, and his best days are the best he's ever had.

Comprehensive Examination

If the screening shows reason for concern, the next step is a comprehensive examination. The form this takes depends on the practitioner since different specialists tend to focus on different physical causes.

In a dental office, we have your child lie back in the dental chair, so we can get a good look at her tongue, tonsils, and adenoids. We'll check her teeth, hard palate, and soft palate as well. We may ask her to demonstrate nasal breathing for us and look for signs of excessive mouth breathing, acid reflux, tooth grinding, or other disorders.

In an ENT office, they may focus more on the tonsils, adenoids, and sinuses. The important thing is that your child receives a comprehensive examination that can identify any potential causes of blocked or restricted airways.

Referrals

After your child's examination, you may receive referrals. For instance, if there appears to be sinus involvement, we may give you a referral to an ENT or allergist. If we suspect your child needs additional testing before we begin treatment, we'll either refer you to a sleep lab or refer you to another practitioner who can refer you to a sleep lab. (The rules on who can refer a patient for a sleep study vary by insurance plan and state. Most practitioners will follow the procedures that get you the best insurance coverage for your child.)

The Sleep Study (and other tests)

The gold standard for diagnosing sleep breathing disorders is a sleep study. In a sleep study, your child spends the night in a hospital sleep lab (with you close by). Their breathing, oxygen levels, heart rate, and brain patterns are monitored to see how they're sleeping, how often they're waking, and whether their body is having trouble getting enough oxygen at night.

Sleep labs often look like hotel rooms. For children, there is usually a bed in the room for an adult companion as well, so you can stay with your child for the test. You'll arrive at the hospital in the evening, go through your child's bedtime routine (snacks, tooth brushing, stories, songs, etc), and then let them fall asleep.

If your child stops breathing or has restricted breathing at all while they sleep, they'll receive a diagnosis of sleep apnea. If your child has no moments where they stop breathing during the test, but you still suspect sleep problems, don't give up. Investigate some of the other Sleep Thieves, and talk to your referring doctor or dentist about next steps. There is help for your kid, and a sleep lab is one of the tests that will help you find the underlying causes of your child's sleep disturbances.

Diagnosis

If the sleep study shows that your child has apneas or hypopneas (that is loss of air or restricted air) during sleep, your child will receive a diagnosis of obstructive sleep apnea, usually from their pediatrician or an ENT. After the diagnosis, it's time for you to consider next steps. There are many treatments for sleep apnea, and you should choose the course of treatment that best addresses your child's underlying issues and that works best for your family.

What are the most common treatments if my child is diagnosed with OSA?

Once your child has been diagnosed with OSA, the treatments open to you depend on other underlying causes. Here are a few of the most common:

Improved Allergy Care. If your child can't breathe through his nose because of swelling and blockage due to allergies, the first line of treatment is often better medications. These can include OTC steroid nose sprays, OTC antihistamines, prescription strength medications, reducing exposure at home, and even allergy shots. If you suspect that allergies are causing your child's issues, ask for a referral to an allergist. Allergy care is generally covered by medical insurance, and it is essential for preventing long-term health issues for your child.

If your child is a mouth-breather, allergies are sometimes to blame. Once you have the allergies under control, you can reestablish nasal breathing and improve sleep breathing.

Tongue and Lip-tie Revision. For a child with tongue-tie and/or lip ties, revising the ties can improve speech, eating, palate development, dental health, and sleep breathing. If your child has underlying ties, it's important to get treatment. Depending on your insurance, these can be a dental expense, a medical expense, or both.

When a newborn needs ties revised, it can happen with a quick procedure in the dental or pediatric office. For children older than a few weeks old, you will need to see an ENT or dentist who specializes in these procedures. Ties can be released either by cutting or with a laser. Your practitioner will choose a method based on your child's age, the location and thickness of the ties, and your family preferences.

After the release procedure, your child will have exercises to do to enhance healing and to ensure that the ties do not reattach. You'll be amazed at what a difference this procedure can make in an older child's life. I've seen children who were told they would never get their "Rs" master this sound in just a month or two after release – they literally couldn't easily move their tongue to make these sounds before. Children who were "chokey" and finicky and who got food stuck in their teeth are suddenly able to chew, swallow, and move food easily around their mouths with just a little instruction. There's a reason that some parents will happily travel 4-6 hours from home to give their children access to this procedure.

Asthma treatments. Sometimes, untreated or undertreated asthma can cause sleep breathing treatments. Often children in their tweens have a "honeymoon period" where their asthma goes into remission for a few years, and then it comes roaring back at puberty. With maintenance inhalers, rescue inhalers, and allergy treatments, you can keep your child's airways open. Either your pediatrician or your allergist should be able to assess your child and provide appropriate medications.

Orofacial Myofunctional Therapy. This branch of occupational and speech therapy focuses on teaching the muscles of the face and mouth to work together. If a child hasn't been using these muscles properly, they need exercises to grow stronger and more coordinated, just like an athlete needs specific exercises to get better at a sport. It's just that in this case, the "sport" is breathing, eating, and speaking.

OMT is especially helpful for children who have either had a tongue tie released or have had severe untreated allergies or speech issues. When a child's tongue is released, they need to practice moving the newly freed tongue, jaws, and cheeks together to support chewing, swallowing, and speaking well. They also need exercises to train their tongue to rest in the palate, not in the middle or bottom of the mouth.

Before a child can position their tongue properly while sleeping, they must be in the habit of positioning it properly while awake.

For habitual mouth-breathers who are now receiving proper allergy treatments, OMT can help reestablish nasal breathing by giving them a series of exercises to practice each day. Just as a speech therapist sends home "homework" like saying the names of particular pictures, an OMT will send home assignments about tongue exercises and nasal breathing.

OMT is important, but it must occur at the right time in treatment. A child whose allergies are still untreated can't learn nasal breathing because their nose is blocked. One whose tongue is still tethered can't learn to move it freely. OMT can work quickly when a child's underlying issues are resolved and the parent and child are faithful about completing exercises.

Many medical insurance plans will cover OMT if there is a documented medical need. Depending on the plan and the state, you may need to go through your child's PCP for treatment. However, most OMTs can help you go through the necessary insurance processes.

Palate expansion. If your child's tongue and lip ties are released before age 2, there is often no need for palate expansion. With practice, their tongue will rest on the roof of the mouth and act as a natural palate expander as they grow, leaving plenty of room for good airflow and proper alignment of permanent teeth.

If, however, your child is older, they may need to have a device called a palatal expander. Palatal expanders help the palate widen and flatten as your child grows. Proper palate shape allows unrestricted nasal breathing, appropriate facial growth and development, easier speech and chewing, proper tooth positioning, and proper tongue position.

To breathe well during sleep, your child needs a palate that both opens up the sinus cavity and that provides a resting place for their tongue. Palate expansion reshapes their palate to support breathing for years to come.

Tonsillectomy and Adenoidectomy. Also called a T&A, this is a surgery that removes your child's tonsils and adenoids. This surgery tends to have few complications in older children and is often the *first* line of treatment that insurers will consider. However, it's important to find root causes after a T&A, or you're setting your child up for a recurrence of OSA as they age and grow.

While swollen tonsils and adenoids do block airways and make breathing harder, often these are swollen as a result of mouth breathing. When the sinuses do not properly filter, humidify, and heat air, breathing irritates and inflames the throat, tonsils, and adenoids.

In addition, mouth breathing means more frequent respiratory infections. Since tonsils and adenoids are one way the body fights off dangerous respiratory viruses and bacteria, they swell when a kid gets sick constantly.

Even if you opt for T&A for OSA treatment, it's important to reestablish nasal breathing and treat any palate deformities, tongue ties, or allergies. Taking care of these issues now can prevent obesity, type 2 diabetes, and heart disease as your child ages.

In the next chapter, we'll look even more closely at how the physiology of the mouth and throat contributes to obstructive sleep apnea, and what you can do to ensure your child gets healthy sleep right now and for the rest of their life.

CHAPTER 6
PALATES, TONGUES, AND TONSILS

In the last chapter, we touched a little on why swollen tonsils and adenoids may be the most obvious cause of an obstructed airway during sleep but not the root cause. In this chapter, we're going to go a little more in-depth. We'll learn more about what the tonsils and adenoids are, what can trigger swelling, and why they sometimes block the airway and trigger apneas (no air) and hypopneas (restricted airflow) during sleep.

WHAT ARE TONSILS AND ADENOIDS ANYWAY?

Your adenoids sit at the top of your throat, where your sinuses connect with the rest of your airway. Your tonsils, meanwhile, are on either side of your mouth. Normally they are so tiny you don't even notice them, but when they swell they feel sore and can temporarily restrict your airways. When you get a sore throat with a cold, it's often because of your swelling tonsils.

Tonsils and adenoids are made of lymphatic tissue. They're an important part of your immune system. These glands trap viruses and bacteria as they enter your body, alerting the rest of the immune system to the attack. White blood cells then learn how to fight the attackers and flood your body, battling the disease and keeping it from hurting you.

These glands are especially important in the first few years of life and keep young children safe from respiratory invaders. Usually, they shrink as a person grows, and they play a less important role in the adult immune system than they do in children.

When your tonsils and adenoids are fighting off diseases, they swell. Normally they return to their normal, nearly invisible. When they're fighting diseases constantly, or if they're irritated and inflamed for other reasons, they can become permanently swollen and impact hearing, breathing, swallowing, and speaking. When this happens, some ENTs recommend a tonsillectomy and adenectomy, or T&A surgery.

What is T&A surgery?

T&A surgery refers to completely removing a person's tonsils and adenoids. If you read older children's books when you were young, characters frequently had their tonsils out. They'd go to the hospital, have surgery, wake up, get presents, and eat nothing but ice cream for a few days. Children's books made T&A surgery look like a lot of fun! The reality of T&A today looks very little like these stories.

While T&A surgery used to be a childhood rite of passage, antibiotics changed the picture. Today, kids don't get chronic bacterial infections that make their tonsils and adenoids swell, because we have antibiotics that treat strep throat and ear infections. When a modern child gets T&A surgery, it's usually as a treatment for obstructive sleep apnea or if their ENT recommends it for other issues.

What happens when a child gets T&A surgery?

Today, most T&A surgeries are outpatient surgeries. When your child has surgery they will:

- Have to arrive with an empty stomach.
- Have an IV placed and monitoring devices attached.
- Undergo general anesthesia (they will be totally asleep, not just sedated.)
- Have the tonsils and adenoids removed via the mouth.
- Wake up in the recovery room.
- Return home with you.
- Need to take a pain killer and eat soft and cool foods for about a week after surgery.

While this is now considered minor surgery, the anesthesia can be a concern, especially for children with certain pre-existing health issues. That means that it is not available to all children with OSA.

Are there any long-term effects of T&A surgery?

For many years, physicians assumed there were no bad effects from this surgery. After all, it had been nearly universal for many decades in the United States. However, in 2018 an international team of researchers completed a huge study of children, following them from their surgery until age 30, and comparing them with control groups who had similar health issues at age 9 but never got surgery. ***It turns out that common knowledge about T&A surgery was wrong.***

The researchers discovered that children who had the surgery had a much higher rate of asthma, allergies, breathing issues, and respiratory infections as adults than children who never had surgery. Even in adulthood, tonsils and adenoids keep working to fight disease. (Chances are if you have yours, you already knew this because they've swollen for you at times.)

Meanwhile, children with the surgery didn't have a significantly lower risk of OSA at 30. The surgery appeared to provide only temporary relief of symptoms.

For parents, this means three things:

1. T&A might still be worth it if your child's symptoms are so extreme that they require immediate relief

2. T&A won't solve the problem permanently. To give your kid healthy sleep and a healthy life, you're going to need to understand why the tonsils and adenoids blocked the airway, and how to solve the underlying health problems that cause the swelling.

3. If it's not an emergency, it may be better to address the swelling of the tonsils and adenoids with other treatments before you choose removal.

WHY DO TONSILS AND ADENOIDS SWELL?

Tonsils and adenoids can swell for two reasons: Because they're working hard, or because they're irritated.

When your child's body is fighting off an invader, their lymphatic tissue swells. Tonsils and adenoids swell if they've inhaled possibly infectious particles such as:

- Bacteria

- Viruses
- Fungal Spores
- Mold and Mildew (and their spores)

Common environmental irritants can also make your child's tonsils and adenoids swell, for instance:

- Smoke – from cigarettes, forest fires, campfires, barbeques
- Allergens like dust, mold, pollen
- Pollution like smog, construction dust, exhaust fumes

When you know why these glands swell, you can try to reduce your child's exposure to irritants and diseases.

How does mouth breathing contribute to swelling?

Mouth breathing contributes to the swelling of tonsils and adenoids because it exposes them to more irritants and invaders than nasal breathing does, and it makes the air itself more irritating to these glands and the entire airway.

Remember, your child's sinuses have several jobs to do:

1. They trap fungus, viruses, and bacteria to give the immune system a head start on fighting them.
2. They filter out particles that could irritate the throat and lungs.
3. They humidify the air to support ease of breathing.
4. They make the air body temperature so that it doesn't irritate the airways.

When a child (or an adult – pay attention to your own breathing too!) bypasses the sinuses, then the air that hits the tonsils and adenoids is:

- Full of viruses and bacteria that need to be caught, identified, and attacked (with swelling glands).
- Full of irritating particles that irritate the lymphatic tissues, throat, and lungs.
- Dry, and prone to dry other tissues out.
- Too hot or too cold, and therefore irritating to the cells in the lymphatic tissues, throat, and lungs.

Mouth breathing makes these glands work overtime while exposing them to a constant stream of irritants that ought to have been filtered out by the nose and sinuses! No wonder they become swollen and painful.

Why is my child a mouth-breather anyway?

Children breathe through their mouths whenever their nose is blocked. If the nose is blocked for too long, mouth breathing becomes a habit. Since "a bad habit is hard to break," once a child has become a mouth breather it takes time and focus to re-establish nasal breathing. And, you won't have any luck re-establishing nasal breathing until you can clear the obstruction.

So, what can cause a long-running blockage in the nose?

Frequent colds and sinus infections

Sometimes a kid gets hit with one cold after another for months at a time, or develops a chronic sinus infection that never gets treated because there's no fever and the child only rarely reports pain. Mouth-breathing becomes a habit.

Injuries

Sometimes, a child will get hit with a ball, get a terrible nosebleed, and then start mouth breathing. Maybe they're just freaked out about the pain and blood from the accident, or maybe they need to be seen to make sure they didn't break anything. No matter what, these kids need support to get comfortable with nasal breathing again.

Deviated Septum

When the wall that divides the nostrils bows to one side or the other, it can block airflow and lead to mouth breathing. This can be a congenital deformity or the result of an injury. Either way, the child needs surgery to fix the septum and restore nasal function.

Allergies

Severe and un- or undertreated allergies can cause chronic blockages in the nose and sinuses. Children with untreated allergies can start mouth-breathing during their peak seasonal allergies and then make it a life-long habit.

A high, arched palate

The roof of the mouth is the floor of the nasal cavity. When it has a high arch, that intrudes into the space where air should flow, making it harder to breathe. Since the space is now unusually narrow, any of the other causes of mouth breathing have a greater chance of restricting airflow to the point where children have to breathe through their mouths to get air.

Swollen adenoids

Wait, isn't this a contradiction? Doesn't mouth breathing cause swollen adenoids? Yes, it does. But then as the adenoids swell, they block off the passage from the nose to the throat, causing even more mouth breathing! This is one reason it can be so hard for a child to break the habit once it starts. Mouth breathing changes the adenoids in ways that make mouth breathing even more comfortable, and the habit solidifies.

An Ounce of Prevention...

For parents, one of the best ways to prevent swollen tonsils and adenoids and the bad effects of OSA is to prevent mouth-breathing in your child, and to take steps to break the habit if you see it happening. ***All children mouth-breathe sometimes***, for instance, after heavy exercise or when they have a bad cold. It only becomes a problem when it becomes a habit that lasts long after it is necessary.

How can you prevent it?

- **Treat colds promptly.** Use natural nose-openers like steam, garlic, or soups to open up those nasal passages and let the nose run. Saline nose spray or neti pots can help wash out stuck secretions. If the natural methods don't work, over-the-counter meds like guaifenesin to thin secretions can be a big help. For smaller kids who are too young to blow their nose, don't forget the magic of the nasal aspirator to clean out the nose and reestablish nasal breathing.

- **Avoid allergens, especially in the sleeping area.** HEPA filters can keep little noses clear at night. If your child has allergies, or is just a generally snotty kid, keeping the night air clear is a high priority. Also, if you suspect allergies, get that kid diagnosed and treated!

- **Remind your kids to sit up straight and breathe right.** One place mouth breathing can become a habit is in front of screens. When kids are sitting slack-jawed and zoned out, they can forget to breathe properly. Be aware, and keep them breathing right.

- **Ask your dentist about habit correctors.** There are soft, rubbery oral appliances that can help younger children learn how to keep their mouths closed and breathe through their noses. These can be a big help to younger kids who are beginning to develop bad habits.

- **Get congenital differences of the palate and tongue treated.** Tongue ties and high palates contribute to nasal blockages and mouth breathing. If your child has issues with either of these, get them treated as young as possible so the sinus cavity can develop!

Evaluate and Treat Tongue-Ties First!

If Tonsillectomy and Adenectomy is the typical first line of treatment for OSA in children, why should you treat tongue tie and related issues first? Because when we treat the underlying cause of the blockage and the swollen glands, many children don't need a T&A after all. They can keep these valuable parts of their immune systems and improve their odds of avoiding OSA as they age. It's a win-win.

So when should you suspect that a tongue-tie might be contributing to your child's problems?

- Your child's siblings, cousins, parents, or aunts and uncles have or had tongue ties. **Tongue-tie often runs in families.**

- Your family has the MTHFR mutation that makes it harder to process folic acid supplements. **Tongue tie is common with this mutation.**

- Your child had other midline deformities, such as spinal cord, heart, or bladder defects at birth. **Tongue-tie is a common midline deformity, and midline deformities often clump together.**

- At birth, the doctor mentioned that your child had a mild tongue-tic, but not serious enough to clip. **The seriousness of a tongue-tie can't always be determined by looking. It depends on how the child reacts to the tongue-tie and how it changes as the child grows.**

- Your child was hard to nurse. They nursed constantly, and it hurt to nurse them. You struggled with blocked ducts and mastitis, but from the outside, the latch looked fine. It might have been so painful and time-consuming that you gave up, even though you wanted to nurse. **Tongue-tied kids are harder to nurse.**

- Your child was gassy and colicky. **Tongue-tie makes swallowing harder, so these kids swallow more air when they nurse or take a bottle.**

- Your child had trouble with the switch to solid food. New foods and textures were hard. They choked a lot. They could handle thin purees and solids like cheerios, but foods in between just made them gag. **Tongue-ties make it** *harder to move solid food around the mouth and swallow. Thicker foods can get packed into the palate and cause gagging.*

- Talking was hard for your child. They were mushy-mouthed and had a hard time making common consonant sounds. *Kids with tongue ties often need speech therapy from a young age.*

- Even as the baby teeth erupted, you could see that your child would need braces someday. *Tongue and lip ties can affect the development of the mouth and palate and the placement of baby and adult teeth.*

- Your child's speech is alright except for certain sounds, especially l,r,t,s, and c. Unfortunately, these sound confusions made phonics and learning to read, a lot harder. *Sounds that require a child to lift the tongue are nearly impossible for some kids with tongue ties. Since they can't make all of the English speech sounds, they have a harder time making the connection between sounds and letters, and between the words on the page and words as they speak them. Your child is a very fussy eater, and still chokes and gags a lot. Certain textures are especially hard, and they always get a lot of food stuck in their teeth. As a result, they are cavity-prone. A child with a tongue tie cannot effectively move food around the mouth or clean food off their teeth with their tongue.*

- Your child has more trouble than their peers do blowing bubbles or blowing up balloons. They may even be unable to blow out birthday candles without spitting or to use a straw appropriately. *Tongue ties can also affect a child's ability to shape their tongue to direct airflow, which keeps them from performing many everyday tasks.*

- Your child's dentist has suggested that there isn't enough room for all of the adult teeth and that healthy adult teeth will need to be pulled to straighten the others. *A tied tongue cannot naturally expand a child's palate into one that can fit all of the adult teeth.*

Tongue ties affect so many aspects of our lives. In fact, many adults with OSA are finding that releasing their tongue ties improves their sleep breathing too! This is why proper evaluation for a tongue tie is a must before you choose a treatment for your child.

Why Can fixing Tongue-Tie Fix OSA?

Releasing a tongue tie can often mean huge changes for kids with OSA. Why? There are a few ways in which a tongue tie contributes to the disease.

It affects the posture of the mouth and jaw. Sit up straight with your mouth closed while practicing good nasal breathing. Where is your tongue? If you don't have a tongue tie, the answer is most likely "On the roof of my mouth.

Now, put your tongue at the bottom of your mouth, so that it rests at the same level as, or even lower than, your teeth. What naturally happens to your mouth? IT OPENS. Tongue tie can cause a slack-jawed posture that makes mouth breathing more likely. If you want to support nasal breathing, you need to make it easier for your child to rest in a close-mouthed position, and that means releasing the tie.

Good tongue position and tone are essential during sleep. When a tongue is tied, it collapsed back in the throat during sleep, restricting the airway. If a child already has swollen tonsils or adenoids, this can tip them over into OSA. One way to train the tongue to keep the airway clear is through a series of exercises that strengthen the tongue muscle and help it support proper nighttime breathing. Guess what kind of tongues are untrainable? Tethered tongues! Releasing the tie makes it possible to resolve a child's issues with orofacial myofunctional therapy (OMT).

What Comes Next after a Tongue-Tie is Released?

In conjunction with the release of a tongue tie, we need to take a two-pronged- approach.

OMT to Support Healthy Habits and Better Breathing

On the one hand, that kid needs OMT as soon as possible. This will teach them how to use their newly freed tongue to speak, eat, and breathe better. In OMT, a child learns a series of exercises to do daily – they don't take long, and they're easy to do while sitting in the car, playing a video game, or waiting in line.

Depending on the child, how much they practice, and how often they can get OMT, there can be a dramatic improvement in as little as 6 weeks. OTs and SLPs may also be able to offer OMT services if there is not a dedicated OMT in your area.

Palate Expansion to Support Proper Breathing

In addition to the therapy to teach the tongue how to move to support speech, eating, and breathing, your child will need some sort of therapy to address the palate issues that come from years with a tongue tie.

Remember, the problems with a tongue tie start in the womb. When a child's tongue can move, it acts as a natural palate expander even before they're born.

Then, as they grow through toddlerhood and early childhood, the tongue helps the palate widen and flatten so that the upper arch of the mouth has room for all of the adult teeth. The expanding palate also opens the sinuses and gives the adult face its shape.

If your child has only recently had a tongue tie released, they've missed out on chances for the palate to flatten during growth spurts. The older they are, the more growth spurts they've missed, and the more help their palate will need to expand.

For toddlers and very young preschoolers, a soft habit corrector may or may not be enough. They have many years of growth ahead of them, and if we can get them used to keeping their tongue in the palate now, there's a good chance they can catch up on lost time.

The older a child (or adult – adults expand their palates too) is, the longer and more intense the expansion process will be. However, you don't want to skip this step. Expanding that palate now protects your child's airway for their entire life.

Get Asthma and Allergies Squared Away

While you're treating the tongue and palate, it's important to get those nasal passages opened up and to keep the lungs open and able to breathe. If you suspect asthma and allergies, you need to get your child treated. Even if you don't currently suspect these disorders, read through the warning signs below. Movies and TV don't always portray these conditions accurately, and even experienced parents can miss the symptoms in their kids.

Your child can have the most mobile tongue or the flattest palate in the world, but if he's struggling with asthma and allergies, those tonsils and adenoids will stay swollen and he won't achieve a clear airway.

- **Asthma isn't always wheezing, and it doesn't always happen with exercise.** The three most common asthma triggers in children are allergies, exercise, and stress (physical or emotional). A child can have all three triggers, or just one. Kids with asthma also aren't all wheezy kids.

If your kid has a nagging cough all night? That's often asthma triggered by allergies. Do you have a drama queen who starts crying, then coughs and throws up? That can be stress-induced asthma.

Does every cold go to "croup" with your kid, even though they're way past the normal croupy age? Asthma. Because asthma tightens the lower airways and makes it hard to breathe, it can make OSA even worse. *Watch for wheezing OR coughing.*

- **Allergies stack.** We're all familiar with what major allergies look like – they're dramatic and involve things like hives, right? But minor allergies can 'stack' and cause big problems too. If your child has many minor allergies but is exposed to all of them all the time, she'll end up with a permanently stuffy nose, weird rashes, breathing issues, and digestive upsets.

This is why allergy testing is so important. Some allergens are easy to eliminate; others are impossible. But by taking out the easiest targets, you can improve your child's overall allergy profile and relieve symptoms.

A fairly easy and common target is dust. You can dust-proof your child's sleeping area and see vast improvements almost instantly. Believe it or not, corn is a tricky one. Why? Because even if you eliminate it from the diet, if you live in much of the country, corn dust is literally in the air at harvest time. You can control your house, but not the great outdoors. Getting an accurate profile gives you and your child more control over allergies and keeps those airways open.

- **Watch out for these signs of allergies and asthma:**
    - *"Raccoon eyes."* Does your child have dark rings around their eyes all the time? This is a tell-tale sign of untreated allergies.
    - *Puffy face in the morning.* Kids with allergies often have swelling around the front of their faces when they wake up in the morning.
    - *Tired, achy, and whiny.* It's not just kids who aren't sleeping who can't function. Kids who can't breathe well during the day also tend to be draggy and cranky. You would be too, if your chest was always tight.
    - *Random coughing fits.* Remember, it's not normal for a kid to have fits of dry coughing all the time. Sometimes I get parents in the office who argue this point because *they* have coughing fits as well. Asthma and allergies run in family. After you get your child screened, make an appointment for any adults with similar issues.
    - *Lots of nosebleeds.* When the nasal tissues are irritated by allergies, they also become more sensitive. Kids with untreated allergies get more nosebleeds than healthy kids.
    - *Frequent stomach pain, vomiting, constipation, or diarrhea.* Some food allergies can affect kids breathing *and* their entire digestive tract. And when kids are allergic to pollen, it can also end up in their stomachs and send things haywire. Plus, when a kid is overwhelmed by one allergy,

say, cedar pollen, other allergens also give stronger reactions, because their body is on high alert.

When you combine allergy and asthma treatment with tongue-tie release, palate expansion, and OMT, most children's adenoids and tonsils can return to normal. They can sleep with an open, functional airway while keeping their upper airway's lymph nodes intact.

WHAT IF WE TRY ALL OF THESE THINGS, AND THE TONSILS AND ADENOIDS ARE STILL A PROBLEM?

Sometimes, even after these less invasive interventions, a kid just has abnormally large tonsils and adenoids. In that case, a T&A can be a good choice. However, the other interventions aren't wasted.

While most kids who get a T&A will redevelop OSA as they age, a kid who has had her tongue tie released, her palate expanded, her allergies and asthma treated, and who has retrained her tongue with OMT *will have a much lower risk of OSA and the conditions that accompany it as she grows older*. These interventions keep her healthy in the long-term, not just during childhood.

CHAPTER 7
SUPPORTING HEALTHY SLEEP AT HOME

Now that you understand the importance of healthy sleep at home, it's time to create a plan to support that sleep. This chapter will teach you the basics of sleep hygiene, while also giving you some tips for changing your family's habits in positive ways for healthy sleep.

Screen Time, and How to Limit It

In an ideal world, all screens would be off after dinner. But in a busy world of kids and activities and jobs and school, this is often an impossible dream. So, aim for no screens for you or your kids an hour before bed.

Sounds great, right? But how can you make that happen?

Baby Steps to Less Blue Light

- **Use Night Mode.** Night mode filters out the blue light so that your phone or computer reducesthe amount of melatonin-disrupting blue light you get before bed. It can take some getting used to, especially if you're watching videos or playing games. However, it does great things for sleep. Schedule night mode to begin at 5 or 6 pm on all of your family's devices, and reduce your evening blue light exposure without having to reduce your screen time.

- **Lock those devices.** Many tablets allow you to lock some apps but not others at night. So, for instance, you can leave homework, music, meditation, and audiobooks unlocked, but lock up the addictive games or the messaging and social media apps that keep your child from winding down to sleep at night. To reduce tantrums, start by locking them at bedtime, and slowly push back the lock time to an hour before bed. *Gradual steps are more effective than sweeping changes that don't stick.*

- **Replace screen time after dinner with other activities.** If you have to work or your child needs screens for homework after dinner, this can be tough. Start with bedtime and work backward. Replace a bedtime cartoon with read-aloud, lullaby, or yoga time. Then, replace "screens during bedtime preparation" with conversation or chores. Slowly eliminate the places where unnecessary screens have worked their way into the bedtime routine. This goes for you, too. Yes, supervising bedtime is boring, but you'll sleep better if you stay off social media and live in the present.

- **If work and homework last until bedtime, reevaluate your life.** We all get busy with sports and activities and end up cramming work and homework into our limited evenings. However, at this time of day, the screens disrupt our sleep and we don't have our best selves to give to work and school. Take a week, and commit to no screen work after dinner (warn your child's teachers.) See if sleep improves. If it does, and if you and your child are waking up refreshed, consider moving that work and homework to the morning when it won't disrupt the brain so much.

- **If you can't go screen-free for an hour, try the last 15 or 30 minutes before bed.** Small steps are still an improvement for your child. Try to get them reading, listening to music, or engaged in prayer/meditation without screens for at least that last 15 minutes to start. Remember, you're not just building a good habit for now, you're helping them build a good habit for life.

What to do About all the CFL and LED Lights

Look around your house. How many of your lights emit mostly blue light? (That's the kind that makes everyone's skin and hair look worse.) How many of those lights are in the sleeping areas? Your lights are impacting your kid's sleep.

Fortunately, amber-colored LED lights are now widely available and affordable. These lights give a warmer light that won't interfere with your child's melatonin production (and makes you look younger and healthier – it's a win for everyone!).

Replacing all the bulbs in the house is expensive so try replacing them in this order:

- Replace any nightlights with amber-light nightlights. Studies have shown that it takes just two blue nightlights in a house to disrupt sleep and cause night-waking.

- Next, do the kids' rooms. Either wait until their lights burn out to replace, or start replacing a few at a time as you can afford to.

- After the kids' rooms, do your room. You also deserve to sleep well.

- For the bathroom, many people like blue light since it makes it easier to examine skin, hair, and teeth (this is why medical examining rooms tend to have blue light). Leave the blue lights in, but use amber nightlights at night so people can use the restroom without being exposed to blue light and waking up.

The kitchen, dining room, and living room are problematic, as you'll want bright light sometimes, and orange light after dinner. Consider investing in smart lightbulbs that will adjust their color according to your needs. These bulbs have also come down in price over the last few years, and are long-lasting LED technology.

Just as with screen time, it's fine to make incremental changes to improve your family's sleep. Just keep moving in the right direction, and you can improve your family's physical, mental, and emotional health!

Steps to Creating Allergy-friendly Sleeping Areas

We've talked a lot about creating allergy-friendly sleeping areas. Here's a step-by-step guide.

1. **Pick up that dirty laundry**! Your kid's dirty laundry should be put in a hamper daily and carried out of the room before bedtime. Because dust mites eat dead skin, laundry is a favorite habitat for them.

2. **Wash the bedding on hot every week.** Yes, this will make it wear out faster. But the cost of the extra laundry is actually far less than the health costs that come from

untreated allergies in the bedroom. Hot water and a hot drier doesn't just remove the dust mite detritus that causes allergies, it kills the mites themselves and gives your child a chance to breathe easier at night.

3. **Invest in dust covers for mattresses and pillows.** These are relatively cheap but provide a huge value since dust mites also love living in pillows and mattresses.

4. **Purchase a HEPA filter.** There are lots of options out there. The low-end ones with replaceable filters work just fine, but you can go for a high-end option if there are other features that you or your child enjoy.

5. **When you can save up the money, replace carpet with laminate, bamboo, wood, or tile.** Carpet is yet another dust mite habitat, which means your family is kicking up allergens into the air every time they take a step. If you *must* have carpet instead of a solid covering, look into lower-pile types like Berber carpet. The thicker and more luxurious the carpet, the better it is at filling up with allergens and the harder it is to get truly clean.

6. **Limit stuffies and pets in the room and on the bed.** Why did I rank this intervention absolutely last? Stuffies are dust mite habitats and pet dander can irritate sleeping noses, but these are also the things kids will kick up the biggest fit about. (Yes, even more than about using a hamper properly). If you can get your kids' allergies under control with the first five interventions, you can let stuffies and pets slide for now.

Foods and Supplements that Support Healthy Sleep

Sleep is a physical process, and every part of our body plays a role in it. If you've ever had indigestion at night, you know that what you eat can play a huge role in your ability to fall asleep and stay asleep all night long. Here are some foods to consider adding you your kids' diet if you want them to sleep well and wake up happy:

Whole grains

It can be hard to make the switch from refined flour to whole grains, but if you can, make the switch from white flour to wheat flour and white rice to brown rice even once or twice a week. Or, if you can't convince the family to switch, at least convince them to try oatmeal made from rolled oats! Why?

Whole grains have more fiber, more vitamins and minerals, and a lower glycemic index than white grains. That means that you:

- Have better digestion and less constipation

- Make more serotonin, a chemical that promotes relaxation at bedtime

- Get more magnesium, a mineral that protects your heart and helps you relax

- Don't have a blood sugar peak and crash. Instead, you have a more level blood sugar and feel full for longer after eating

When your kids eat whole grains, they'll feel satisfied, relaxed, and sleepy all night, and get better sleep while improving their whole-body health.

Healthy fats

A totally fat-free diet is bad for the brain and bad for sleep. Without enough fat, people get depressed and anxious. Their body thinks there must be a famine in the land, so they wake up a lot at night, always hungry and desperate for food. Healthy fats, especially Omega-3 fatty acids, improve sleep. For healthy sources of dietary fat try:

- **Fatty fish like salmon and mackerel** – These are rich in Omega-3 fatty acids
- **Nuts and seeds** – Nuts and seeds are great sources of healthy fats if your child isn't allergic. Many are also natural sources of melatonin and great sources of protein. Plus, they're foods that level out blood sugar and keep kids feeling full. If allergies aren't a problem, walnuts, almonds, sesame seeds, pumpkin seeds, peanuts and soy all belong in your child's diet.

Choose the right fruits and veggies

- **Kiwis** contain serotonin, which involved in making melatonin. Since melatonin plays an important role in both falling asleep and staying asleep, kiwis can be a great addition to your child's diet.
- **Tart Cherries** contain both serotonin and melatonin. Consider adding them to dessert time for a better night's sleep.
- **Broccoli** is a superfood. It doesn't just contain important nutrients like magnesium and potassium. It's also a natural source of melatonin! Include it in your day as much as possible.

Supplements that impact sleep

Nutritional deficiencies can have a huge, negative impact on sleep. And for many busy families with finicky kids, it can be tough to eat a balanced diet. Here are supplements that can help with sleep:

- **Omega-3 Fatty Acids.** Omega-3 fatty acids are important for mood, memory, and sleep. Free range eggs and fatty fish are good sources, but there are also supplements available.

- **Iron.** Low iron is linked to poor sleep at night and exhaustion during the day. If your kid is fussy about nuts, beans, and meat, they may end up needing a supplement.

- **Magnesium.** Does your family love nuts, seeds, beans and leafy greens? If not, it may be time for a magnesium supplement. Magnesium supports a healthy cardiovascular system and promotes sleep.

- **Potassium.** Low potassium is another common problem in kids who don't eat a ton of fruit. If your kid hates oranges and bananas, they may need a boost of this nutrient.

- **L-methyl folate.** There's a growing body of evidence that this particular form of folic acid can improve mood and sleep, even in people who don't have a genetic reason for taking it.

- **Melatonin.** Some kids are genuinely low melatonin, and supplements can get them to go to sleep. Unfortunately, there are no extended-release versions currently available in the US, which means they may have trouble STAYING asleep, but it's a start.

Reset your kid's circadian rhythm

We all feel terrible when we get off schedule, but there are ways to reset circadian rhythms and get your kid back on schedule.

- **Get out and see the sun (or lack thereof).** Sunlight tells our body when to wake and when to sleep. Make sure your kid gets both mid-day and evening sun so that their body knows what time it is.

- **Eat dinner as a family and wind down together.** Social signals have a strong effect on circadian rhythms – our brains want us to be in sync with the people we love. Meanwhile, when someone is alone on a screen for hours, their brain can lose track of the meaning of time. So spend time together, yawn together, and help your kid's brain get the social cues that tell them bedtime is soon.

- **Wake up earlier and run them hard.** It can be tough to make sure your kids get enough exercise during the school week, but on weekends, try to wake them up at their normal school time, and then wear them out during the day so that falling asleep is easier. This can retrain the brain.

The best exercises for sleep

Aerobic exercise pumps you up. It can relieve stress and help you sleep later, but it takes a while for the endorphins produced to wear off so you can calm down for sleep. Experts recommend stopping aerobic exercise 1-2 hours before sleep.

Weight lifting and yoga also improve sleep, as long as you do them for at least 30 minutes a day.

Many people find bedtime yoga routines can help them wind down, calm their minds, and get to sleep at night.

Breathing exercises are an excellent way to prepare for sleep. Try breathing the square, where you breathe in for 4 beats, out for 4 beats, in for 4 beats, out for 4 beats. Teach your child to do this too, in order to relax muscles and lower blood pressure for sleep.

DESTRESS BEFORE BEDTIME

Stress affects kids more than we like to admit, and many kids need bedtime rituals to help them release the stress of the day and embrace calm and rest. Different kids need different destressing techniques. You may need to experiment to find out what helps your kid unwind. Some possibilities are:

- A read aloud or a book on tape
- Favorite music
- White noise
- A hot bath
- Time to talk
- Time to journal
- Cuddles
- Tickles
- Warm drinks (Caffeine-free, of course)
- A night-time walk
- An open window
- Time to draw or read
- Practicing an instrument

- Prayer
- Meditation

Every kid is different and every kid has different needs. Find out how to help yours destress and put the worries of the day aside so that they can get the sleep they need.

What about bedwetting?

Bedwetting is a huge sleep stealer, even when it's not caused by sleep apnea. The discomfort and shame can make a kid hate going to sleep and hate waking up.

There are a few things you can do to reduce bedwetting and improve your child's sleep:

- **No drinks 2 hours before bed.** Some kids just have immature bladders that need more time to grow.

- **Triple void before going to sleep.** Make sure your children start the night with an empty bladder.

- **Up the fiber.** Bedwetting can be a sign of chronic constipation. Make sure your child is getting enough whole grains, fruits, and veggies

- **Test for UTIs**. Bedwetting in the absence of OSA can also be a sign of chronic UTIs. Talk to your doctor about having your child's urine tested.

- **Consider a bedwetting alarm.** Some children don't have enough Phase 2 sleep at night to recognize when they have to get up and go. A bedwetting alarm can retrain their brains. (For the first few weeks the alarm is more for the parent than the child).

- **Ask your doctor about next steps.** If your child is 10 or 11 and still wetting the bed nightly and does not appear to have sleep apnea, it might be time to see a specialist. Talk to your doctor about what to do next and what referrals you'll need.

- **Be positive and supportive!** Your child is more embarrassed and upset by this than you are. Try to support them and respect them as you sort out this medical issue.

We were doing great—until we hit the teens!

I don't know a single parent who's happy with how their teens sleep. The combination of shifted circadian rhythms, heavy homework loads, phones, and friends means that our teens are going to bed much to late to survive their early school starts.

With teens, you have less control over sleep habits. This is a time of life when they need to start taking charge of their own health, so they're ready to launch in a few years. Still, there are a few things you can do to help them get more sleep and to prepare them to respect their health as they mature.

- **Get that phone charger out of the bedroom.** If your kid can charge their phone in bed, they can be on their phone in bed. Keep the chargers in public areas so that it's easier for your kid to detach from the phone at bedtime.

- **Check on them when you go to bed.** Yes, your teen may be up late working on homework, but even a reminder that they should at least shower, put on PJs, and wind down can help them get to sleep. Sometimes they just *forget*, and you can be their brain.

- **Let them sleep in as late as possible in the morning.** School starts too early for teens. Help them in their efforts to make mornings more efficient so that they can get the most sleep possible.

- **Keep an eye out for anxiety and depression.** Teens have it rough, and mental illness is on the rise. 17% of teens struggle with depression and 31% have anxiety. Lack of sleep may contribute, but mental illness steals sleep. A good therapist can help your kid work through their feelings and get better sleep at night.

- **Lock down the wifi after midnight.** This can keep kids from getting too sucked into online games. Once they can't game or watch TV, they might go to bed.

- **Talk to your teens about healthy sleep and why sleep is important.** Yes, they'll ignore you right now, but in a few years they'll remember and start taking your advice.

- **Don't let sleep fights ruin your relationship.** They will grow out of this stage, and they will eventually start loving sleep again, as we all do once we're out of the house and out in the world. If your otherwise healthy kid is staying up too late, it's OK to let go a little, especially if their mood and grades are fine.

Teenagers often push their bodies to the limit, and their bodies' limits are much further out there than their parents' are. Your kid is growing up so fast. Help them towards healthy sleep, but not at the risk of enjoying these last few years with them at home.

Dr. Meghna Dassani

YOU'RE WELL ON YOUR WAY TO GREAT SLEEP FOR YOUR KIDS

If you can put even a fraction of these lists to use, your kids will be in great shape when it comes to sleep!

Remember, healthy sleep is great for the whole family, not just your kids. Create a family culture of healthy sleep, and you'll all feel happier, more energetic, and ready to take on the world!

CHAPTER 8
CONGRATULATIONS! YOU'RE A KIDS' SLEEP EXPERT

Have you worked your way through this whole book? Do you understand the signs of a kid who isn't sleeping well and who might need a sleep evaluation? Have you identified the sleep stealers in your own home?

Congratulations! You know more about sleep than many medical professionals, and you're ready to advocate for your own children, and the children of friends and family members. Sleep is the foundation of health, learning, and social skills. When you spread the word about healthy sleep in your community, you save futures and even lives.

It's time for moms to stop being shy about offering advice and supporting each other in their children's sleep journeys. When you see a mom whose child is a mouth-breather, or who is tired and draggy, or who is a whirlwind of impulse and emotion, ***she already knows there is something wrong with her child.***

What she might not know is where to start, or who can help. Once you've had a kid or two go through sleep screenings, tongue tie release, or OMT to support good breathing and tongue position, you *do* know where to find help. Talk to people. Listen to their worries. Be the person who can offer connections and solutions, not just criticism. Once you've been there with your own kids, you can support other families who need to learn about sleep, airways, and breathing.

I firmly believe that when we correct a child's sleep problems, we change their life. We give them a future where they can breathe, sleep, learn, make friends, and dream big. So reach out. Build a community of airway experts. Share this book with your friends, family, your children's teachers and health providers. Start a movement, and start saving lives.

Meghna Dassani DMD

APPENDIX 1
RESOURCES FOR FINDING HELP FOR YOUR CHILD

Do you need to…

Find a pediatric ENT? Try The American Society of Pediatric Otolaryngology's page at: **https://aspo.us/page/findanent**

Find a sleep lab? Try the American Academy of Sleep Medicine's page at: **https://sleepeducation.org/sleep-center/**

Find an Orofacial myofunctional therapist? Try the Academy of Orofacial Myofunctional Therapy at: **https://aomtinfo.org/find-a-therapist-2/**

Find a speech and language pathologist? Try the American Speech-Language-Hearing Association: **https://www.asha.org/profind/**

For dentists willing to release tongue and lip ties, lactation consultants can be a great resource, as can speech pathologists, La Leche league, and OMTs. Professionals in your region work together and can help you find someone who will take your concerns seriously.

You can always ask your family dentist or pediatrician about a sleep screening. If your dentist doesn't have a pediatric sleep dentistry program, they may know someone nearby who does!

Local social media groups and parenting groups are another great source of provider recommendations. People love to share what helped their own kids. Someone will know about a provider who can help you.

Most of all, don't give up. Help is out there. Keep pushing, keep asking, and eventually you will find the provider who is willing to change your child's life.

APPENDIX 2
BOOK CLUB DISCUSSION GUIDE

Introduction and Chapter 1

1. Why did you pick up this book? Who are you reading it for?

2. Do you have any children in your personal or professional life who have some of the symptoms of a child with sleep problems?

3. What surprised you most in Chapter 1? Did you learn anything new?

4. Imagine yourself as a sleepless child. You're sitting in a first grade desk, and the teacher has just handed out a timed test. How do you feel? What do you say? What do you do? What could the adult present do to help you through this pain?

5. If you have a child who has some of these symptoms, what are three things you hope for their future self?

6. What are three things you fear for their future self?

7. What can you do to help them grow up healthy and strong?

Chapter 2

1. Think about your family. Who are the early birds? Who are night owls? What sort of jobs are best for early birds? Where can night owls really soar?

2. Do you have any funny stories to share about people you've known with odd sleep hours?

3. Do you remember your dreams? Have there been times in your life when you didn't?

4. Do you wear a sleep tracker? What do you notice about your deep and light sleep patterns? Have you ever tried having your child wear it for a night or two? How were their patterns different from yours? (If you haven't tried this yet, will you try it this week and report back at the next group meeting?

5. What was the most interesting thing you learned about sleep in this chapter? How will you apply it in your life or your kids' lives?

Chapter 3

1. Which sleep thieves are especially familiar to you? How do they affect your family?

2. Have you noticed any signs of sleep apnea in your kids?

3. When was the last time you talked to a doctor about sleep? What did they say?

4. Is there one sleep thief you can try to eliminate this month?

CHAPTER 4

1. Do you suspect someone in your family might have airway problems? Why? What have you noticed?

2. What facts about the airway are new and exciting for you? Which were old news?

3. What's your favorite home remedy for keeping sinuses open? Will your kids go along with it or do they complain?

4. Now that you know about tongue and jaw position, do you find yourself changing yours?

5. What signs of a restricted airway are you going to look for in your family?

6. If you're out and meet a mother whose child seems to have airway issues, what will you do next?

CHAPTER 5

1. Look back at the list of providers in the chapter. How many of these do you have in your life? Do you know anyone with good recommendations? Share your recommendations with the group and discuss.

2. Has anyone ever screened your child for sleep issues? When?

3. Who will you ask to screen your child at their next appointment? The pediatrician? A dentist?

4. Record your child's breathing for a bit some night. What do you notice?

CHAPTER 6

1. Why might it be a bad idea to make T&A the first line of treatment for pediatric OSA?

2. Does your child have any signs of tongue tie?

3. Rest and breathe with your tongue in the roof of your mouth and your lips sealed closed. Now, try to breath when your mouth is open and your tongue rests in the bottom of your mouth. Which is more comfortable? Which makes it easier to breathe? Which is more calming?

4. Do you know any children with undertreated asthma and allergies? Do you have undertreated asthma and allergies? (Hint: if you frequently can feel your lungs or find in effortful to breathe, see your doctor)

5. How could changing how a child breathes change their life?

CHAPTER 7

1. Take another look at the lists of ways to support healthy sleep at home. Pick 4. Try to add one each week for the next month. Which 4 did you choose?

2. Which tips sound like fun? Which sound like something you could never see your family doing?

3. Who is the worst sleeper in your house? Which tip could help them the most?

4. Pick one tip, as a group, to try to implement in your homes. Be each other's accountability partners.

5. When you were a teen and a college student, what was your sleep like? Are your teens better or worse than you were? What's the craziest young adult sleep story you have?

Chapter 8

1. How are you going to change lives with everything you've learned?

2. Who will you share this book with next?

APPENDIX 3
SOURCES AND FURTHER READING

ARTICLES

Chapter 1

Kean, Nikki. "The Dramatic Rise in Tongue Tie and Lip Tie Treatment". *ENTToday.* Sept 6, 2019.
https://www.enttoday.org/article/explaining-the-dramatic-rise-in-tongue-tie-and-lip-tie-treatment/?singlepage=1

Segal, Lauren M., Stephenson, Randolph., et al. "Prevalence, diagnosis and treatment of Ankyloglossia." *Canadian Family Physician.* June, 2007.
https://www.ncbi.nlm.nih.gov/pmc/articles/PMC1949218/

Chapter 2

Anrillon, Thomas., Nir, Yuval., et al. "Sleep Spindles in Humans: Insights from Intracranial EEG and Unit Recordings." *Journal of Neuroscience.* Dec 7, 2011
https://www.ncbi.nlm.nih.gov/pmc/articles/PMC3270580/#:~:text=Sleep%20spindles%20are%20an%20electroencephalographic,memory%20consolidation%20to%20cortical%20development.

Gagnon, Katia., Bolduc, Christianne., et al. "REM Sleep EEG Activity and Clinical Correlates in Adults with Autism." *Frontiers in Psychiatry.* June 8, 2021
https://www.ncbi.nlm.nih.gov/pmc/articles/PMC8217632/

Chapter 3

Danner, Fred and Phillips, Barbara. "Adolescent Sleep, School Start Times, and Teen Motor Vehicle Crashes." *Journal of Clinical Sleep Medicine.* December 15, 2008.
https://www.ncbi.nlm.nih.gov/pmc/articles/PMC2603528/

Chapter 6

Byars, Sean G., Stearns, Stephen C., et al. "Association of Long-Term Risk of Respiratory, Allergic and Infectious Diseases with Removal of Adenoids and Tonsils in Childhood." *Journal of the American Medical Association Otolaryngology – Head and Neck Surgery.* July, 2018.
https://jamanetwork.com/journals/jamaotolaryngology/article-abstract/2683621

Chapter 7

"Exercising for Better Sleep." *Health*. Johns Hopkins Medicine.
https://www.hopkinsmedicine.org/health/wellness-and-prevention/exercising-for-better-sleep

Cronkleton, Emily. "8 Stretches to do before bed." *Healthline*. Feb 5, 2021
https://www.healthline.com/health/stretching-before-bed

"How Box Breathing Can Help You Destress." *Health Essentials*. Cleveland Clinic. August 17, 2021
https://health.clevelandclinic.org/box-breathing-benefits/

OTHER READING:

Walker, Matthew. *Why We Sleep: Unlocking the Power of Sleep and Dreams*. Scribner, New York: 2018

Dassani, Meghna. *Airway is Life: Waking up to your family's sleep crisis*. 2021

Ehlin, Carl-Joan Forssen. *The Rabbit Who Wants to Fall Asleep: A New Way of Getting Children to Sleep*. Crown, New York: 2014

Gates, Mariam. *Goodnight Yoga: A Pose-by-Pose Bedtime Story*. Sounds True: 2015.

APPENDIX 4
WORKSHEETS

My Healthy Sleep Plan

My Name is _____

I am _____ Years old so I need _____ hours of healthy sleep a night.

I need to be up at _____ so I will go to bed at _____ every night.

Since I am going to bed at _____ I will turn off all my screens by _____.

My Bedtime routine:
1.
2.
3.
4.
5.

To relax and fall asleep I can:
1.
2.
3.
4.

Some healthy bedtime snacks I like are:
1.
2.
3.

My Sleep Team

Provider	Phone/Email
Dentist:	
Pediatrician:	
SLP:	
OMT:	
ENT:	
Sleep Lab:	
Pharmacy:	
OT:	
PT:	
Other:	

Made in the USA
Coppell, TX
18 September 2025